Current Cardiovascular Therapy

Gheorghe-Andrei Dan
Antoni Bayés de Luna
John Camm
Editors

Juan Carlos Kaski
Series Editor

Atrial Fibrillation Therapy

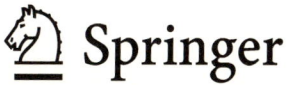 Springer

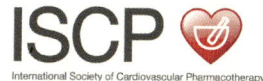
International Society of Cardiovascular Pharmacotherapy

Editors

Gheorghe-Andrei Dan, MD PhD, FESC, FAHA
Internal Medicine Clinic and Department of Cardiology
Colentina University Hospital
Bucharest
Romania

Department of Internal Medicine and Cardiology
Faculty of Medicine
University of Medicine and Pharmacy Carol Davila
Bucharest
Romania

Antoni Bayés de Luna, MD FESC, FACC
The Catalan Institute of Cardiovascular Sciences
Hospital Santa Creu i Sant Pau
Barcelona, Spain

John Camm, MD, FRCP(London), FRCP(Edin), FACC, FESC, FMedSci, FHRS, CStJ
Cardiovascular Sciences Research Centre
Division of Clinical Sciences
St George's University of London
London, United Kingdom

ISBN 978-1-4471-5474-7   ISBN 978-1-4471-5475-4   (eBook)
DOI 10.1007/978-1-4471-5475-4
Springer London Heidelberg New York Dordrecht

Library of Congress Control Number: 2013955577

© Springer-Verlag London 2014
This work is subject to copyright. All rights are reserved by the Publisher, whether the whole or part of the material is concerned, specifically the rights of translation, reprinting, reuse of illustrations, recitation, broadcasting, reproduction on microfilms or in any other physical way, and transmission or information storage and retrieval, electronic adaptation, computer software, or by similar or dissimilar methodology now known or hereafter developed. Exempted from this legal reservation are brief excerpts in connection with reviews or scholarly analysis or material supplied specifically for the purpose of being entered and executed on a computer system, for exclusive use by the purchaser of the work. Duplication of this publication or parts thereof is permitted only under the provisions of the Copyright Law of the Publisher's location, in its current version, and permission for use must always be obtained from Springer. Permissions for use may be obtained through RightsLink at the Copyright Clearance Center. Violations are liable to prosecution under the respective Copyright Law.
The use of general descriptive names, registered names, trademarks, service marks, etc. in this publication does not imply, even in the absence of a specific statement, that such names are exempt from the relevant protective laws and regulations and therefore free for general use.
While the advice and information in this book are believed to be true and accurate at the date of publication, neither the authors nor the editors nor the publisher can accept any legal responsibility for any errors or omissions that may be made. The publisher makes no warranty, express or implied, with respect to the material contained herein.

Printed on acid-free paper

Springer is part of Springer Science+Business Media (www.springer.com)

Series Preface

Cardiovascular pharmacotherapy is of fundamental importance for the successful management of patients with cardiovascular diseases. Appropriate therapeutic decisions require a proper understanding of the disease and a thorough knowledge of the pharmacological agents available for clinical use. The issue is complicated by the existence of large numbers of agents with subtle differences in their mode of action and efficacy and the existence of national and international guidelines, which sometimes fail to deliver a clear-cut message. Aggressive marketing techniques from pharma industry; financial issues at local, regional, or national levels; and time constraints make it difficult for the practitioner to – at times – be absolutely certain as to whether drug selection is absolutely appropriate. The International Society of Cardiovascular Pharmacotherapy (ISCP) aims at supporting evidence-based, rational pharmacotherapy worldwide. This book series represents one of its vital educational tools. The books in this series aim at contributing independent, balanced, and sound information to help the busy practitioner to identify the appropriate pharmacological tools and to deliver rational therapies. Topics in the series include all major cardiovascular scenarios, and the books are edited and authored by experts in their fields. The books are intended for a wide range of healthcare professionals and particularly for younger consultants and physicians in training. All aspects of pharmacotherapy are tackled in the series in a concise and practical fashion. The books in this series provide a unique set of guidelines and examples that will prove valuable for patient management. They clearly articulate many of the dilemmas clinicians face when working to deliver sound therapies to their patients. The series will most certainly be a useful reference for those seeking to deliver evidence-based, practical, and successful cardiovascular pharmacotherapy.

Juan Carlos Kaski, DSc, DM (Hons),
MD, FRCP, FESC, FACC, FAHA

Preface

Atrial fibrillation has been the low man on the totem pole and so we're just trying to get more visibility about this particular disease and how dangerous this could be (Barry Manilow, American singer)

Atrial Fibrillation (AF) has a long history, but in many regards it remains a challenging *terra incognita*. In the oldest medical text written earlier than 400 B.C., the Chinese "Yellow Emperor's Inner Canon" (or better Huang Di Nei Jing Su Wen), we find the following quotation: "*When the pulse is irregular and tremulous and the beats occur at intervals, then the impulse of life fades; when the pulse is slender (smaller than feeble, but still perceptible, thin like a silk thread), then the impulse of life is small.*" Much later, in the seventeenth century, it was William Harvey who rediscovered and described the arrhythmia in dogs, but the first electrical characterization was done during the mid-nineteenth century by the French Felix Alfred Vulpian who also baptized the disease "*fremissement fibrillaire.*" Other nicknames were "*pulsus irregularis perpetuus*" (Hering) or even more suggestive "*delirium cordis*" (Cushny). Two Austrian doctors, Rothberger and Winterberg, identify "arrhythmia perpetua" as being atrial fibrillation. Shortly after the invention of the electrocardiogram by Einthoven, it was Sir Thomas Lewis to send to his Dutch friend the first tracing from a patient with atrial fibrillation. The mechanism of atrial fibrillation was a longtime subject of debate (and this debate still continues). After Sir Thomas Lewis and his pupil C. C. Iliescu stated that reentry is the main mechanism of AF and atrial flutter, it was Scherf to propose the automaticity as the main mechanism and the reentry as a consequence. Ten years later, Moe put the basis for the multiple wavelets theory, and the reentrant theory dominated our understanding of the AF mechanism. Although initially considered mutually exclusive, we know now, after the discovery by Haissaguerre of the role of pulmonary foci in triggering AF, that reentry and focal triggering mechanisms are complementary in the mechanisms of AF initiation and perpetuation. After Bouilland discovered that digitalis may reduce the heart rate in AF (without abolishing irregularity) and Bootsma revealed by means of a computer modeling that the mechanism of random concealed conduction of atrial impulses within the AV node is responsible for an irregular ventricular rate, it was only during the late 1960's when Lown recommended cardioversion of AF. After 1980, the Framingham study emphasized the link between AF and stroke and on prognostic implications of this arrhythmia. We know now that AF became an epidemic disease because of aging population and because of increase in the prevalence of chronic heart disease and risk factors. By 2050 as many as 30 million may suffer from this disease. Overall, the mortality for patients with AF is double that in patients in sinus rhythm, and the divergence in the survival curves was noted from the moment of AF diagnosis. The most important contributor to the worse outcome in patients with AF is represented by the ischemic stroke, five times more prevalent in patients with AF and carrying the worst mortality and functional impact among all ischemic strokes. There are several accepted pharmacologic management strategies in AF: prevention of atrial remodeling or reverse remodeling (upstream therapy), systemic embolism prevention, and arrhythmia therapy (heart rate control and/or rhythm control including conversion to sinus rhythm and prevention of recurrences). The aim of therapy is to improve survival and quality of life, to improve symptoms, to reduce consequences (stroke, embolism, or heart failure), to reduce hospitalizations, to restore atrial function (reverse remodeling), and to minimize the adverse effects of medication. Despite huge progress made in understanding mechanisms responsible for initiation and perpetuation of atrial fibrillation and of complex pathophysiology of this complex disease, the actual treatment of AF is far from being perfect. The same is true about the awareness of the disease impact among medical and patient milieu. Refinement in the research of the subtle molecular targets for newer and safer antiarrhythmics, new diagnostic tools for revealing global AF burden, establishing better targets of primary prophylaxis, and further progress in interventional therapy (ablation) will improve the management and the outcome of AF. Ablation of AF (through removal of triggers and substrate modification) improved substantially the management of AF. However, at least at this moment, AF ablation cannot be seen as a substitute of the pharmacologic therapy. Prevention of ischemic stroke in AF patients with oral anticoagulants represents a huge challenge, and the enormous amount of research is revealing new treatment opportunities at a dizzying pace. A new era has begun for the prevention of stroke, one of the most devastating complications of AF. While new classes of antithrombotic drugs for AF treatment are still in their infancy, recent research is revealing how these can be applied with optimal efficacy in clinical practice.

The present book, *Atrial Fibrillation Therapy*, includes practical information for readers on applying the guidelines developed as a result of the increased pharmacotherapeutic understanding. This book also aims to guide trainees, recertifying physicians, and practicing physicians in internal medicine, cardiology, emergency medicine, and clinical pharmacology to apply the new diagnostic tools for selecting the best treatment options for AF patients. The intention of the authors is more to discuss and emphasize the current aspects of AF therapy than to draw definite conclusions because, as was once said, "*drawing definite conclusions means that the author became too tired to think.*"

Gheorghe-Andrei Dan
Antoni Bayés de Luna
John Camm

Contents

Contributors List

Cristian Baicus, MD, PhD Carol Davila University of Medicine and Pharmacy Bucharest, Bucharest, Romania

Department of Internal Medicine, Colentina University Hospital Bucharest, Bucharest, Romania

Gheorghe-Andrei Dan, MD, PhD, FESC, FAHA University of Medicine "Carol Davila", Bucharest, Romania

Internal Medicine Clinic, Cardiology Department, Colentina University Hospital, Bucharest, Romania

Dan Dobreanu, MD, PhD Department of Physiology and Institute of Cardiovascular Disease and Transplant, University of Medicine and Pharmacy of Tîrgu Mures, Tîrgu Mures, Romania

Yuri Gluzman Heart Institute, Edith Wolfson Medical Center, Holon, Israel

Sackler Faculty of Medicine, Tel-Aviv University, Tel Aviv, Israel

Antoni Bayés de Luna, MD, FESC, FACC Catalan Institute of Cardiovascular Sciences, Hospital Santa Creu i Sant Pau, Barcelona, Spain

Antoni Martínez-Rubio, MD, PhD, FESC, FACC Department of Cardiology, University Hospital of Sabadell, Sabadell, Barcelona, Spain

Yoseph Rozenman, MSc, MD, FACC Heart Institute, Edith Wolfson Medical Center, Holon, Israel

Sackler Faculty of Medicine, Tel-Aviv University, Tel Aviv, Israel

Alina Scridon, MD, PhD Department of Physiology and Institute of Cardiovascular Disease and Transplant, University of Medicine and Pharmacy of Tîrgu Mures, Tîrgu Mures, Romania

Josep Guindo Soldevila, MD Cardiology Service, Hospital Parc Tauli de Sabadell, Sabadell, Barcelona, Spain

Chapter 1
Epidemiology, Burden and Unmet Needs in Atrial Fibrillation

Antoni Martínez-Rubio, Josep Guindo Soldevila, and Antoni Bayés de Luna

Introduction

Atrial fibrillation (AF) is an arrhythmia characterized by chaotic electrical activity in the atria, which causes asynchrony of atrial fibers excitation and contraction. Thus, the organized contractile capacity of the atrium for filling the ventricles is lost which diminishes the ventricular ejection, as well as auricular blood stasis and turbulent flow favors thrombosis and consequently thromboembolism may develop. Therefore, this arrhythmia has an important clinical impact. This chapter summarizes the several unmet needs in AF, which still constitutes a challenge for patients, physicians and health care managers because its medical, social and economic impact probably will worsen over the next decades. Therefore, research and future knowledge of AF will play a major role for modern societies.

A. Martínez-Rubio, MD, PhD, FESC, FACC (✉)
Department of Cardiology, University Hospital of Sabadell,
Parc Taulí s/n, E-08208 Sabadell, Barcelona, Spain
e-mail: 22917amr@comb.cat

J.G. Soldevila, MD
Cardiology Service, Hospital Parc Tauli de Sabadell, Sabadell,
Barcelona, Spain

A.B. de Luna, MD, FESC, FACC
Catalan Institute of Cardiovascular Sciences,
Hospital Santa Creu i Sant Pau, Barcelona, Spain

G.-A. Dan et al. (eds.), *Atrial Fibrillation Therapy*, Current
Cardiovascular Therapy, DOI 10.1007/978-1-4471-5475-4_1,
© Springer-Verlag London 2014

Epidemiology

AF affects 1–2 % of the population with incremental incidence and prevalence in relation to age [1]. The projected estimations predict and increase (at least doubling) of affected individuals during the next 30 years [2, 3]. Furthermore, recent studies show that approximately 6 % of patients attended primary care physicians [1] and 31 % of hospitalized patients in Internal Medicine and Geriatric wards [4] present AF. In addition, AF is the first cause (47 % of attended patients) of anticoagulation in Hematological Departments [5]. Thus, the first unmet need of AF management is the lack of epidemiological control of AF incidence and prevalence (Table 1.1).

Several epidemiological studies have demonstrated that AF increases 2–6 times the probability of suffering a stroke and 1.5–2.2 times the mortality [6–12] (Fig. 1.1). This arrhythmia has been also associated with cognitive dysfunction, diminished quality of life and diminished functional capacity [13–16]. Patients affected of AF often present other comorbidities, which are summarized in Table 1.2 and need specific treatment [6, 10, 15, 16].

Thus, it is obvious that AF is a very often arrhythmia, with increasing numbers of affected persons that consumes a broad portion of the health care resources because it causes complex disabling status, such as ischemic or hemorrhagic stroke [14, 17] and increases mortality. In consequence, the major Cardiology Societies have published guidelines and updates for the management of AF [13, 15, 18–22]. These are extended recommendations, which reflect the broad complexity of clinical manifestations and the difficulties of management. Furthermore, although several concordant aspects between international guidelines exist, there are also some differences in the strategies and even in the available therapies (such as drugs) between different guidelines and different countries. The lack of agreement in some aspects of these guidelines constitutes a challenge for physicians and reflects that several aspects are unresolved in AF.

TABLE 1.1 Unmet needs for the management of atrial fibrillation

Epidemiological aspects

  Lack of epidemiological control of AF

  Comorbidities with unsatisfactory control

  Discrepancies between different guidelines

Antiarrhythmic aspects

  Cardioversion does not preclude recurrence

  Antiarrhythmic drugs have unpredictable effects on the arrhythmia

  Antiarrhythmic drugs have potential side-effects

  Limited number of antiarrhythmic drugs

  Catheter ablation has individually unpredictable long-term effects on the arrhythmia

  Catheter ablation might trigger complications inherent to invasive procedures

  There is no capacity for universal coverage for AF-ablation

  The best method for catheter ablation has not been established yet

  Surgical ablation is invasive and does not either represent an universally available alternative

  Left atrial appendage closure is invasive and does not cure the arrhythmia

Antithrombotic aspects

  Different societies recommend different thromboembolism risk scores

  Diverse bleeding risk scores exists

  Limited data of some populations (e.g. severe renal failure patients are often excluded of trials) exist

  Dicumarine derivates present several limitations for clinical use

  There is a lack of data using the new anticoagulant drugs in some groups of patients (e.g. in patients with acute coronary syndromes)

  No specific antidotes are available for the new anticoagulant drugs yet

  Left atrial appendage is not the only site of thrombus formation

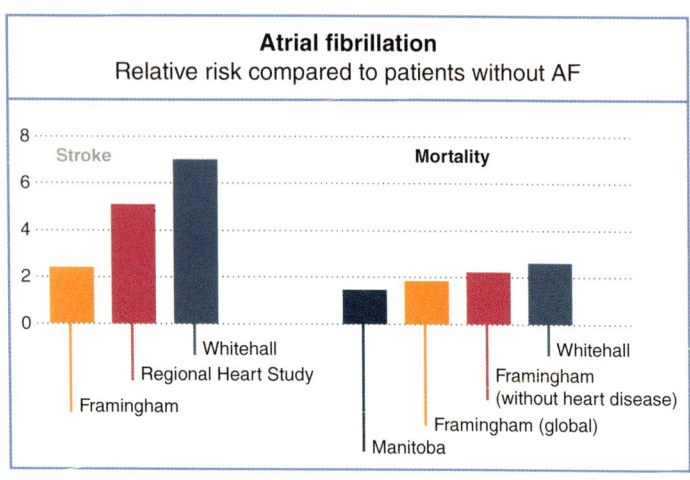

FIGURE 1.1 Relative risk of stroke and mortality of patients with versus without atrial fibrillation in epidemiological studies

TABLE 1.2 Comorbidities associated with high prevalence of atrial fibrillation

Arterial hypertension
Heart failure
Valvular disease
Myocardiopathies (including ischemic heart disease)
Congenital heart disease (i.e. interatrial shunt)
Thyroid dysfunction
Obesity
Diabetes mellitus
Chronic obstructive pulmonary disease
Sleep apnea syndrome
Chronic renal disease
Genetic predisposition

TABLE 1.3 European Heart Rhythm Association classification of symptoms of atrial fibrillation

EHRA I: without symptoms
EHRA II: mild symptoms which do not impair the normal daily activities
EHRA III: sever symptoms affecting normal daily activities
EHRA IV: disabling symptoms impeding normal daily activities

Diagnosis

AF can be suspected by the presence of irregular pulse, but its presence must be confirmed electrocardiographically by:

(a) Absence of P waves replaced by chaotic electrical contractions of the auricular myocites.
(b) Irregular RR intervals caused by variable AV node conduction.

AF usually begins by short and infrequent paroxysmal episodes. With the lapse of time these episodes tend to occur more often and to be longer. Thus, AF episodes trigger electrical and mechanical remodeling, which favors the perpetuation of the arrhythmia.

Symptoms of the arrhythmia may not be present or disabling. The European Heart Rhythm Association has proposed a classification of the perceived AF symptoms (Table 1.3). Unfortunately, those individuals without any subjective symptom, who do not know that they present AF, might suffer complications of AF (e.g. ischemic stroke) as the first manifestation, which may lead to diagnosis of the underlying affection. The most recent guidelines of the European Society of Cardiology recommend opportunistic screening for AF patients ≥65 years of age using pulse-taking followed by an ECG to allow timely detection of AF [19]. Anamnesis of AF is not specific. However, it is very relevant because some patients develop AF related to specific situations (such as after alcohol intake) or have a genetic background [23].

Thus, the recognition of AF triggered by anamnesis is crucial for proper management [24].

Antiarrhythmic Therapies

Being AF a potentially very dangerous arrhythmia, it seems logical to use antiarrhythmic strategies to avoid, or at least control, this rhythm disturbance. The first antiarrhythmic step is "prevention" of the occurrence of the arrhythmia. However, this goal is by far not achieved, as reflected by the increasing numbers of affected individuals. The broad identified numbers of comorbidities associated with increased AF-prevalence (Table 1.2) as well as increasing age of the populations reflect the complexity of a preventive strategy. Clearly, there is no unique necessary strategy but a broad strategy involving each of the identified AF-favoring elements is mandatory.

When a patient develops AF, there are short-term strategies for reversion of the arrhythmia. These are pharmacological and electrical cardioversion. The last consists of an electrical resynchronization of auricular fibers by an energy artificial dipole, which usually is applied externally (transthoracic) with a cardioverter-defibrillator by means of a DC-shock. Although these electric cardioversion is highly effective in the acute setting of AF, this technique does not preclude the recurrence (even short-term recurrence) of AF.

Antiarrhythmic drugs for reversion of the arrhythmia (e.g. flecainide, propafenone, vernakalant, amiodarone, etc.) may be effective, but (a) it can not be individually predicted the effectiveness rate, which highly depends on AF-duration and the underlying heart disease, (b) have potential side-effects (e.g. proarrhythmia) and (c) do not guaranty avoidance of AF-recurrence. Long-term AF-management with antiarrhythmic drugs may, obviously, be also related with side-effects (potentially lethal) and either precludes recurrences. In addition, we have a very limited number of antiarrhythmic drugs clinically available, especially in some subsets of patients (e.g.

heart failure). Amiodarone still remains the best drug to prevent recurrences.

Recently, Tsadok et al. [25] analyzed prescription and follow-up data of 57,518 patients with AF. They reported that in comparison with rate control therapy (n = 41,193), the use of rhythm control therapy (n = 16,325) was associated with lower rates of stroke/transient ischemic attack (TIA), in particular, among those patients with moderate and high risk of stroke. The crude stroke/TIA incidence rate was 1.74 versus 2.49, per 100 person-years (p < 0.001), respectively. This observation was documented although treatment with any antithrombotic drug was comparable in the two groups (76.8 % in rhythm control versus 77.8 % in rate control group).

Cather ablation, with a variety of variant approaches, has been proposed as a curative technique. This strategy has the inherent risk of invasive procedures (e.g. perforation of cavities, embolism, etc.) and it is costly (in short term perspective). Major complications as stroke (0.6 %), tamponade (1.3 %), peripheral vascular complications (1.3 %) and pericarditis (2 %) have been reported from voluntary high-volume centers in the EURObservational Research Programme [26]. Several other centers have also reported complications of the technique [27, 28]. Thus, true complications rates might be even higher. Silent cerebral infarctions have been reported from 4 % to 35 % [29–31]. From a meta-analysis of 4,156 patients, it has been reported a complication rate of 5 % and a rate of all-cause hospitalization in the first year after catheter ablation of 38.5 % [28]. Thus, catheter ablation is a curative approach with inherent risks that should be balanced against more conservative strategies on an individual basis and after detailed information to the patient.

In addition, long-term efficacy of catheter ablation cannot, either, be predicted in an individual basis [32–35]. Unfortunately, several patients will develop short and long-term recurrences after apparently successful ablation [32–35]. Furthermore, although may be a curative solution for selected individuals, universal coverage is impossible at this moment. The very broad number of affected individuals and the limited number of Electrophysiology laboratories that could try to cure AF-patients justifies this affirmation. The randomized MANTRA-PAF trial compared catheter ablation of AF versus antiarrhythmic drug therapy as first-line rhythm control strategy [36]. Catheter ablation was superior for preventing symptomatic AF at 1 and 2 years of follow-up. In addition, those patients of the ablation group reported better quality of life. However, total burden of AF was not significantly different between both subsets of patients [36]. Similar results have been presented by other authors [37].

Surgical ablation seems more effective than catheter ablation but with the cost of a higher complication rate [38]. Therefore, it is a technique reserved for selected patients undergoing other concomitant surgical procedures such as aorto-coronary bypass or valve replacement. Thus, surgical AF-ablation may not be considered a realistic solution for the broad majority of patients affected by this arrhythmia. In consequence, antiarrhythmic drugs, catheter and surgical ablation do not properly solve the clinical impact of AF and constitute several of the unmet needs of AF management (Table 1.1).

Antithrombotic Therapy

Being the actual antiarrhythmic strategies imperfect and of limited clinical value for the eradication of AF, the vast majority of patients will need sooner or later therapy for the prevention of thromboembolism. Thus, oral anticoagulation is a crucial consideration that must be done in all patients suffering of AF. Since antithrombotic drugs increase the probability of bleeding, both risks should be balanced prior to deciding therapy. Several cohort studies have identified different thromboembolic risk factors [6, 10, 39, 40]. With these, different risk scores for thromboembolism have been proposed. Actually, the CHA_2DS_2-VASC is the recommended score [19, 41] for thromboembolism by the European Society

Risk scores in atrial fibrillation			
For thromboembolism: CHA2DS2-VASC		**For bleeding: HAS-BLED**	
CHA$_2$DS$_2$-VASc criteria	**Score**	**HAS-BLED risk criteria**	**Score**
Congestive heart failure/ left ventricular dysfunction	1	Hypertension	1
Hypertension	1	Abnormal renal or liver function (1 point each)	1 or 2
Age ≥ 75 yrs	2		
Diabetes mellitus	1	Stroke	1
Stroke/transient ischaemic attack/Thromboembolism	2	Bleeding	1
Vascular disease (prior myocardial infarction, peripheral artery disease or aortic plaque)	1	Labile INRs	1
Age 65–74 yrs	1	Elderly (e.g. age >65 yrs)	1
Sex category (i.e. female gender)	1	Drugs or alcohol (1 point each)	1 or 2

FIGURE 1.2 Risk scores recommended by the European Society of Cardiology

of Cardiology (Fig. 1.2). However, other major Cardiology Societies recommend the use of other scores. The CHA$_2$DS$_2$-VASC score includes Congestive heart failure/left ventricular dysfunction, Hypertension, Age >75 (doubled), Diabetes, Stroke (doubled), Vascular disease, Age 65–74 years, and Sex category (female). With the CHA$_2$DS$_2$-VASC, it must be remarked that antithrombotic therapy is not recommended in patients with AF (irrespective of gender) who are aged <65 and lone AF (i.e. truly low-risk patients). Heart failure per se is not defined as a risk factor. Thus, the "C" in the CHA$_2$DS$_2$-VASC refers to documented moderate-to-severe systolic dysfunction (i.e. heart failure with reduced ejection fraction) or patients with recent decompensated heart failure requiring hospitalization, irrespective of ejection fraction (i.e. both heart failure with reduced and with preserved ejection fraction). Female gender independently increases the risk of stroke overall, unless the criterion of age <65 and lone AF is clearly fulfilled, whereby female gender does not independently increase stroke risk. Thus, female patients with gender alone as a single risk factor (still CHA_2DS_2-VASC score of 1) would not need anticoagulation if they clearly fulfil the criteria of age <65 and lone AF.

Furthermore, bleeding risk must be also considered prior to anticoagulant therapy and three different scores have been proposed and evaluated in AF patients [42–44]. The European Society of Cardiology suggests the use of the HAS-BLED score (Fig. 1.2) [43] rather than more complicated ore less practical score [19]. This includes Hypertension, Abnormal renal/liver function, Stroke, Bleeding history or predisposition, Labile INR, Elderly (e.g. age >65, frailty, etc.), Drugs/alcohol concomitantly. However, HAS-BLED score does not include some parameters (e.g. cancer, plaquetopenia or altered platelet function) as suggested by other scores [42, 44]. Every score has obviously limitations and different predictive values. In addition, some populations have been practically excluded from clinical trials and therefore, the actual knowledge cannot be surely inferred to such patients (e.g. severe renal failure patients are often excluded from clinical trials).

The most recent recommendations for anticoagulation in AF from the European Society of Cardiology are [19]:

(a) Patients with valvular AF (rheumatic valvular disease (predominantly mitral stenosis) or prosthetic heart valves) should always be anticoagulated (actually with vitamin-K antagonists)
(b) Patients with non-valvular heart disease:

   a. <65 years and lone AF (including females) should not receive antithrombotic therapy
   b. >65 years and/or not lone AF should be assessed by CHAD2DS2-VASc score

      i. If score equals 0 they should not receive antithrombotic therapy.
      ii. If score is one anticoagulant therapy should be considered based upon an assessment of bleeding risk

(HAS-BLED score) and patient values and preferences.

iii. If score is ≥2 antithrombotic therapy is recommended, unless contraindicated.

Because antiplatelet therapy is less effective than antithrombotic drugs for stroke prevention but it presents a similar bleeding risk, antiplatelet drugs are not recommended as first line-therapy in new AF-guidelines [19].

Dicumarine derivatives have been very useful drugs during decades for reducing thromboembolism since they reduce relative risk of stroke about 64 % and of mortality about 26 % versus placebo [45]. In patients treated with these drugs, an International Normalized Ratio (INR) of 2–3, which critically determines the consecutive risk of bleeding, achieves the optimal therapeutic range. Thus, INR >3 increases bleeding risk (especially intracranial bleeding) without significant antithrombotic benefit [15, 46]. However, bleeding may also occur in patients in therapeutic range [47]. In addition, bleeding risk with aspirin is considered to be similar to that with dicumarine derivatives particularly in older persons [19]. The broad number of limitations of dicumarine drugs is summarized in Fig. 1.3.

The new anticoagulant drugs (dabigatran, rivaroxaban and apixaban) are similar o more effective than warfarin to reduce stroke and systemic embolism [48–50] (Fig. 1.4). In addition, these drugs achieve a consistent relative risk reduction of mortality close to 10 % versus warfarin (Table 1.4). In addition, they are able to reduce critical bleeding (such as intracranial bleeding) (Fig. 1.5). The net clinical benefit of the new anticoagulants has been modeled considering stroke and bleeding rates versus dicumarin derivatives [51]. At a CHA2DS2-VASc score of 1, both doses of dabigatran (110 mg b.i.d. and 150 mg b.i.d.) and apixaban had a positive net clinical benefit. All three new anticoagulants (dabigatran, rivaroxaban and apixaban) are superior (in clinical net benefit) to warfarin in patients with a CHA2DS2-VASc score of ≥ 2, irrespective of bleeding risk [51]. Therefore, the European Society of Cardiology guidelines now recommend the new

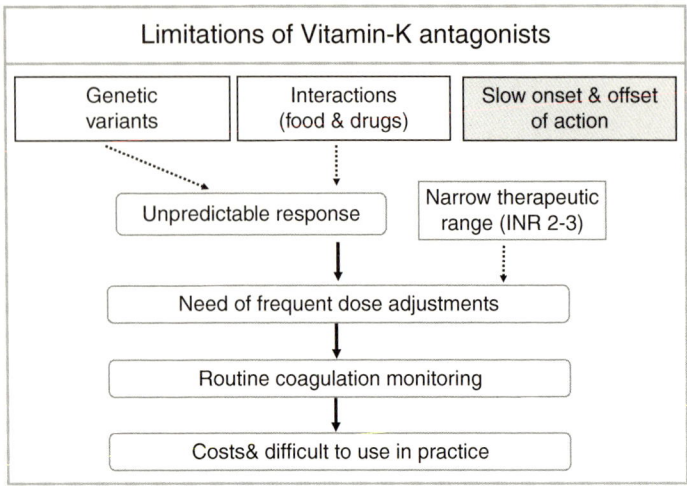

FIGURE 1.3 Clinical limitations of dicumarine derivatives

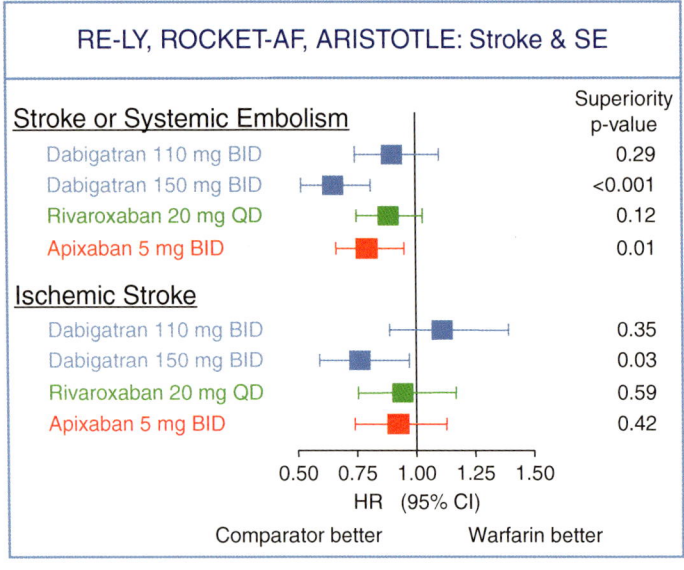

FIGURE 1.4 Stroke and systemic embolism with the new anticoagulants compared to warfarin

New anticoagulants: All cause mortality			
RELY		**RR**	**P-value**
Dabigatran 110 mg	3.75% / yr	0.91	0.13
Dabigatran 150 mg	3.64% / yr	0.88	0.051
Warfarin	4.13% / yr		
ROCKET-AF			
Rivaroxaban 20 mg	1.9% / yr	0.85	0.07
Warfarin	2.2% / yr		
ARISTOTLE			
Apixaban 5 mg	3.52% / yr	0.89	0.048
Warfarin	3.94% / yr		

TABLE 1.4 Reduction of mortality with new anticoagulant drugs compared to warfarin

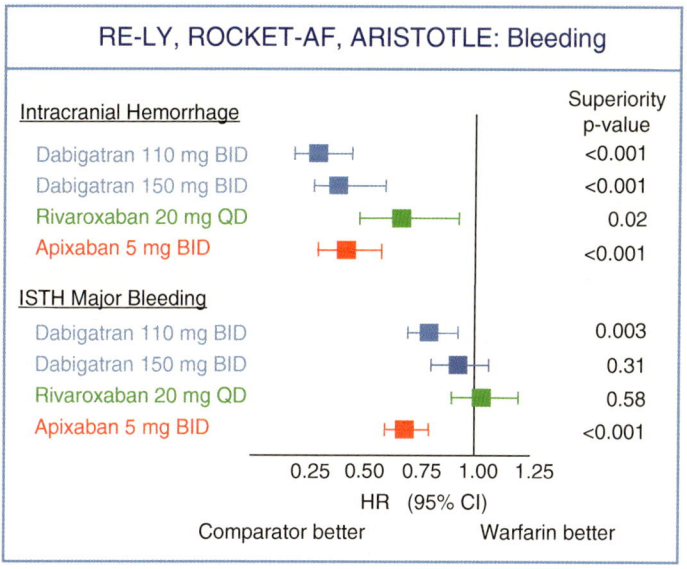

FIGURE 1.5 Bleeding with the new anticoagulants compared to warfarin

anticoagulants over vitamin-K antagonist in the vast majority of patients with non-valvular AF (when used as studied in the clinical trials).

However, actually, there is a lack of data with the use of these drugs in some groups of patients. This affirmation is justified since patients with severe renal failure or with mechanical valves have been excluded from the clinical trials with these drugs. In addition, the benefit/risk profile of the combination of antithrombotic (dicumarinic or new) drugs and dual antiplatelet therapy is not well defined by clinical trials yet [52, 53]. Guidelines recommend that patients with atrial fibrillation (treated with vitamin K antagonists), who present with an acute coronary syndrome or who undergo a percutaneous coronary revascularization, should receive triple therapy (both vitamin K antagonists and dual antiplatelet therapy) [54]. However, recent data demonstrate that triple antithrombotic therapy is associated with early, higher risk of serious bleeding, determining hospitalization or death in comparison with the use of antiplatelets or a vitamin K antagonist alone or the combination of this last drugs with just one antiplatelet agent [55].

Perioperative management with these drugs is still challenging by limited experience for the vast majority of physicians, although the rapid onset and offset of action of these new drugs demonstrates a favorable profile versus vitamin-K antagonists. These very effective drugs for thromboembolism prevention do not have specific antidotes yet, although they are under development. Furthermore, they do not need routinely monitoring of effects, which is an improvement over dicumarine derivates. Some coagulation tests have been proposed for facilitation of decisions during emergencies, but these tests are not universally available yet, although intense research is being performed and, probably, it will not constitute a clinical issue in the very near future.

In spite that the price of the new antithrombotic agents is most expensive, the global cost of the treatment with these drugs versus treatment with warfarin has been analyzed in different countries and situations. The results suggest that already commercially available drugs (dabigatran and rivaroxaban) may be a cost-effective alternative to adjusted-dose warfarin for stroke prevention in AF [56–61].

The precise indications and limitations of use of classical and new anticoagulant drugs are extensively reviewed in other chapters of this book.

Left atrial appendage closure or excision is an alternative for patients at high risk of stroke who present contraindications for chronic oral anticoagulation. However, both techniques are obviously invasive and left atrial appendage is considered the main but not the only site of thrombus formation. Therefore, it cannot be expected that it will prevent all strokes. In addition, the limited experience and evidence of efficacy and safety is insufficient for considering as a universal alternative.

Conclusions

Atrial fibrillation is a growing cardiovascular disease that increases morbidity and mortality originating a first level health challenge for patients, physicians, and health care managers.

Patients suffer directly the morbidity (e.g. stroke, heart failure) and mortality, as well as impaired quality of life. For physicians, AF is a difficult to treat condition (often not curable) without fully satisfactory treatment options. For payers, AF raises de risk of hospitalization and the derivate costs, as well as the cost of side effects and monitoring needed with the existing agents.

Current therapeutic options aim mainly to relieve symptoms and only achieve poor results. The existing antiarrhythmic drugs are associated with toxicities and do not relevantly improve clinical outcomes. There is a need for atrium-selective effective and safe antiarrhythmic drugs. Invasive curative approaches are expanding and might change the scenario. However, universal coverage is unlikely and several open questions remain with these techniques. Thus, the broad

majority of patients will need chronic anticoagulation therapy, which improves outcomes, but must be balanced against
bleeding risk. Antivitamin-K drugs present diverse limitations for use in clinical practice. The new anticoagulants represent an important therapeutic progress, but some open
questions remain to be answered. Dabigatran, rivaroxaban
and apixaban have already demonstrated their clinical utility
in clinical studies. The role of several other new anticoagulants is still in evaluation process.

Thus, AF management has still several unmet needs
(Table 1.1) that have been exposed and deserve further
research and resources.

References

1. Barrios V, Calderón A, Escobar C, de la Figuera M; en represent-
   ación del Grupo de Atención Primaria de la sección de Cardiología
   Clínica de la Sociedad Española de Cardiología. Patients with atrial
   fibrilladion in a primary care setting: Val-FAAP Study. Rev Esp
   Cardiol. 2012;65(1):47–53.
2. Go AS, Hylek EM, Phillips KA, et al. Prevalence of diagnosed atrial
   fibrillation in adults: national implications for rhythm management
   and stroke prevention: the Anticoagulation and Risk Factors in
   Atrial Fibrillation (ATRIA) study. JAMA. 2001;285:2370–5.
3. Miyasaka Y, Barnes ME, Gersh BJ, Cha SS, Bailey KR, Abhayaratna
   WP, Seward JB, Tsang TS. Secular trends in incidence of atrial fibrillation in Olmsted County, Minnesota, 1980 to 2000, and implications
   on the projections for future prevalence. Circulation. 2006;114(2):
   119–25.
4. López Soto A, Formiga F, Bosch X, García Alegría J; en represent-
   ación de los investigadores del estudio ESFINGE. Prevalence of
   atrial fibrillation and related factors in hospitalizad old patients:
   ESFINGE study. Med Clin (Barc). 2011:138(6):231–7.
5. Navarro JL, Cesar JM, Fernández MA, Fontcuberta J, Reverter JC,
   Gol-Freixa J. Morbidity and mortality in patients treated with oral
   anticoagulants. Rev Esp Cardiol. 2007;60(12):1226–32.
6. Atrial Fibrillation Investigators. Risk factors for stroke and efficacy
   of antithrombotic therapy in atrial fibrillation. Analysis of pooled
   data from five randomized controlled trials. Arch Intern Med.
   1994;154:1449–57.
7. Flegel KM, Shipley MJ, Rose G. Risk of stroke in non-rheumatic
   atrial fibrillation. Lancet. 1987;1(8537):526–9.

8. Krahn AD, Manfreda J, Tate RB, Mathewson FA, Cuddy TE. The natural history of atrial fibrillation: incidence, risk factors, and prognosis in the Manitoba follow-up study. Am J Med. 1995;98: 476–84.

9. Benjamin E, Wolff P, D'Agostino R, Silbershatz H, Kannel W, Levy D. Impact of atrial fibrillation on the risk of death: the Framingham Heart Study. Circulation. 1998;98:946–52.

10. Stewart S, Hart CL, Hole DJ, McMurray JJ. A population-based study of the long-term risks associated with atrial fibrillation: 20-year follow-up of the Renfrew/Paisley study. Am J Med. 2002;113(5):359–64.

11. Vidaillet H, Granada JF, Chyou PH, Maassen K, Ortiz M, Pulido JN, et al. A population-based study of mortality among patients with atrial fibrillation or flutter. Am J Med. 2002;113:365–70.

12. Benjamin E, Levy D, Vaziri S, D'Agostino R, Belanger A, Wolf P. Independent risk factors for atrial fibrillation in a population-based cohort. JAMA. 2004;271:840–4.

13. Fuster V, Rydén LE, Cannom DS, et al. ACC/AHA/ESC 2006 guidelines for the management of patients with atrial fibrillation – executive summary: a report of the American College of Cardiology/ American Heart Association Task Force on Practice Guidelines and the European Society of Cardiology Committee for Practice Guidelines (Writing Committee to Revise the 2001 Guidelines for the Management of Patients with atrial fibrillation). Eur Heart J. 2006;27:1979–2030.

14. Kelly-Hayes M, Beiser A, Kase CS, Scaramucci A, D'Agostino RB, Wolf PA. The influence of gender and age on disability following ischemic stroke: the Framingham study. J Stroke Cerebrovasc Dis. 2003;12(3):119–26.

15. Camm JA, Kirchhof P, Lip GYH, Schotten U, Savelieva I, Ernst S, Van Gelder IC, Al-Attar N, Hindricks G, Prendergast B, Heidbuchel H, Alfieri O, Angelini A, Atar D, Colonna P, DeCaterina R, DeSutter J, Goette A, Gorenek B, Heldal M, Hohnloser SH, Kolh P, LeHeuzey JY, Ponikowski P, Rutten FR. Guidelines for the management of atrial fibrillation. Eur Heart J. 2010;31:2369–429.

16. Knecht S, Oelschlager C, Duning T, Lohmann H, Albers J, Stehling C, Heindel W, Breithardt G, Berger K, Ringelstein EB, Kirchhof P, Wersching H. Atrial fibrillation in stroke-free patients is associated with memory impairment and hippocampal atrophy. Eur Heart J. 2008;29:2125–32.

17. Lin HJ, Wolf PA, Kelly-Hayes M, Beiser AS, Kase CS, Benjamin EJ, D'Agostino RB. Stroke severity in atrial fibrillation. The Framingham Study. Stroke. 1996;27:1760–4.

18. Fuster V, Rydén LE, Cannom DS, Crijns HJ, Curtis AB, Ellenbogen KA, Halperin JL, Kay GN, Le Huezey JY, Lowe JE, Olsson SB, Prystowsky EN, Tamargo JL, Wann LS. 2011 ACCF/AHA/HRS focused updates incorporated into the ACC/AHA/ESC 2006

Guidelines for the management of patients with atrial fibrillation: a report of the American College of Cardiology Foundation/American Heart Association Task Force on Practice Guidelines developed in partnership with the European Society of Cardiology and in collaboration with the European Heart Rhythm Association and the Heart Rhythm Society. J Am Coll Cardiol. 2011;57(11):e101–9.

19. Camm AJ, Lip GYH, De Caterina R, Savelieva I, Atar D, Hohnloser SH, Hindricks G, Kirchhof P. 2012 focused update of the ESC Guidelines for the management of atrial fibrillation. Eur Heart J. 2012. doi:10.1093/eurheartj/ehs253.

20. Wann LS, Curtis AB, Ellenbogen KA, Estes NA 3rd, Ezekowitz MD, Jackman WM, January CT, Lowe JE, Page RL, Slotwiner DJ, Stevenson WG, Tracy CM, Fuster V, Rydén LE, Cannom DS, Crijns HJ, Curtis AB, Ellenbogen KA, Halperin JL, Kay GN, Le Heuzey JY, Lowe JE, Olsson SB, Prystowsky EN, Tamargo JL, Wann LS, Jacobs AK, Anderson JL, Albert N, Creager MA, Ettinger SM, Guyton RA, Halperin JL, Hochman JS, Kushner FG, Ohman EM, Stevenson WG, Yancy CW; American College of Cardiology Foundation/American Heart Association Task Force. 2011 ACCF/AHA/HRS focused update on the management of patients with atrial fibrillation (update on dabigatran). A report of the American College of Cardiology Foundation/American Heart Association Task Force on Practice Guidelines. Circulation 2011;123:1144–50.

21. You JJ, Singer DE, Howard PA, Lane DA, Eckman MH, Fang MC, Hylek EM, Schulman S, Go AS, Hughes M, Spencer FA, Manning WJ, Halperin JL, Lip GY; American College of Chest Physicians. Antithrombotic therapy for atrial fibrillation: antithrombotic therapy and prevention of thrombosis, 9th ed: American College of Chest Physicians Evidence-Based Clinical Practice Guidelines. Chest 2012;141:e531S–75.

22. Skanes AC, Healey JS, Cairns JA, Dorian P, Gillis AM, McMurtry MS, Mitchell LB, Verma A, Nattel S; Canadian Cardiovascular Society Atrial Fibrillation Guidelines Committee. Focused 2012 update of the Canadian Cardiovascular Society Atrial Fibrillation Guidelines: recommendations for stroke prevention and rate/rhythm control. Can J Cardiol. 2012;28:125–36.

23. Campuzano O, Brugada R. Genetics of familial atrial fibrillation. Europace. 2009;11(10):1267–71.

24. Bayés de Luna A. Clinical arrhythmology. Wiley-Blackwell; 2011.

25. Tsadok MA, Jackevicius CA, Essebag V, Eisenberg MJ, Rahme E, Humphries KH, Tu JV, Behlouli H, Pilote L. Rhythm versus rate control therapy and subsequent stroke or transient ischemic attack in patients with atrial fibrillation. Circulation. 2012;126:2680–7.

26. Arbelo E, Brugada J, Hindricks G, Maggioni A, Tavazzi L, Vardas P, Anselme F, Inama G, Jais P, Kalarus Z, Kautzner J, Lewalter T, Mairesse G, Perez-Villacastin J, Riahi S, Taborsky M, Theodorakis G,

Trines S; on behalf of the Atrial Fibrillation Ablation Pilot Study Investigators. ESC-EURObservational research programme: the atrial fibrillation ablation pilot study, conducted by the European Heart Rhythm Association. Europace 2012;14:1094–103.

27. Cappato R, Calkins H, Chen SA, Davies W, Iesaka Y, Kalman J, Kim YH, Klein G, Natale A, Packer D, Skanes A, Ambrogi F, Biganzoli E. Updated worldwide survey on the methods, efficacy, and safety of catheter ablation for human atrial fibrillation. Circ Arrhythm Electrophysiol. 2010;3:32–8.

28. Shah RU, Freeman JV, Shilane D, Wang PJ, Go AS, Hlatky MA. Procedural complications, rehospitalizations, and repeat procedures after catheter ablation for atrial fibrillation. J Am Coll Cardiol. 2012;59:143–9.

29. Herrera Siklódy C, Deneke T, Hocini M, Lehrmann H, Shin DI, Miyazaki S, Henschke S, Fluegel P, Schiebeling-Römer J, Bansmann PM, Bourdias T, Dousset V, Haïssaguerre M, Arentz T. Incidence of asymptomatic intracranial embolic events after pulmonary vein isolation: comparison of different atrial fibrillation ablation technologies in a multicenter study. J Am Coll Cardiol. 2011;58:681–8.

30. Di Biase L, Burkhardt JD, Mohanty P, Sanchez J, Horton R, Gallinghouse GJ, Lakkireddy D, Verma A, Khaykin Y, Hongo R, Hao S, Beheiry S, Pelargonio G, Dello Russo A, Casella M, Santarelli P, Santangeli P, Wang P, Al-Ahmad A, Patel D, Themistoclakis S, Bonso A, Rossillo A, Corrado A, Raviele A, Cummings JE, Schweikert RA, Lewis WR, Natale A. Periprocedural stroke and management of major bleeding complications in patients undergoing catheter ablation of atrial fibrillation: the impact of periprocedural therapeutic international normalized ratio. Circulation. 2010;121:2550–6.

31. Gaita F, Leclercq JF, Schumacher B, Scaglione M, Toso E, Halimi F, Schade A, Froehner S, Ziegler V, Sergi D, Cesarani F, Blandino A. Incidence of silent cerebral thromboembolic lesions after atrial fibrillation ablation may change according to technology used: comparison of irrigated radiofrequency, multipolar nonirrigated catheter and cryoballoon. J Cardiovasc Electrophysiol. 2011;22:961–8.

32. Ouyang F, Tilz R, Chun J, Schmidt B, Wissner E, Zerm T, Neven K, Ko¨ktu¨rk B, Konstantinidou M, Metzner A, Fuernkranz A, Kuck KH. Long-term results of catheter ablation in paroxysmal atrial fibrillation: lessons from a 5-year follow- up. Circulation. 2010;122:2368–77.

33. Tzou WS, Marchlinski FE, Zado ES, Lin D, Dixit S, Callans DJ, Cooper JM, Bala R, Garcia F, Hutchinson MD, Riley MP, Verdino R, Gerstenfeld EP. Long-term outcome after successful catheter ablation of atrial fibrillation. Circ Arrhythm Electrophysiol. 2010;3:237–42.

34. Arya A, Hindricks G, Sommer P, Huo Y, Bollmann A, Gaspar T, Bode K, Husser D, Kottkamp H, Piorkowski C. Long-term results and the predictors of outcome of catheter ablation of atrial fibrillation using steerable sheath catheter navigation after single procedure in 674 patients. Europace. 2010;12:173–80.

35. Weerasooriya R, Khairy P, Litalien J, Macle L, Hocini M, Sacher F, Lellouche N, Knecht S, Wright M, Nault I, Miyazaki S, Scavee C, Clementy J, Haissaguerre M, Jais P. Catheter ablation for atrial fibrillation: are results maintained at 5 years of follow-up? J Am Coll Cardiol. 2011;57:160–6.

36. Cosedis Nielsen J, Johannessen A, Raatikainen P, Hindricks G, Walfridsson H, Kongstad O, Pehrson S, Englund A, Hartikainen J, Mortensen LS, Hansen PS. A randomized comparison of radiofrequency ablation and antiarrhythmia drug therapy as first line treatment in paroxysmal atrial fibrillation. N Engl J Med. 2012;367(17): 1587–95.

37. Wazni OM, Marrouche NF, Martin DO, Verma A, Bhargava M, Saliba W, Bash D, Schweikert R, Brachmann J, Gunther J, Gutleben K, Pisano E, Potenza D, Fanelli R, Raviele A, Themistoclakis S, Rossillo A, Bonso A, Natale A. Radiofrequency ablation vs antiarrhythmic drugs as firstline treatment of symptomatic atrial fibrillation: a randomized trial. JAMA. 2005;293:2634–40.

38. Boersma LV, Castella M, van Boven W, Berruezo A, Yilmaz A, Nadal M, Sandoval E, Calvo N, Brugada J, Kelder J, Wijffels M, Mont L. Atrial fibrillation catheter ablation vs. surgical ablation treatment (FAST): a 2-center randomized clinical trial. Circulation. 2012;125:23–30.

39. Stroke in AF Working Group. Independent predictors of stroke in patients with atrial fibrillation: a systematic review. Neurology. 2007;69:546–54.

40. Hughes M, Lip GY. Stroke and thromboembolism in atrial fibrillation: a systematic review of stroke risk factors, risk stratification schema and cost effectiveness data. Thromb Haemost. 2008;99: 295–304.

41. Lip GY, Nieuwlaat R, Pisters R, Lane DA, Crijns HJ. Refining clinical risk stratification for predicting stroke and thromboembolism in atrial fibrillation using a novel risk factor-based approach: the Euro Heart Survey on atrial fibrillation. Chest. 2010;137:263–72.

42. Gage BF, Yan Y, Milligan PE, Waterman AD, Culverhouse R, Rich MW, Radford MJ. Clinical classification schemes for predicting hemorrhage: results from the National Registry of Atrial Fibrillation (NRAF). Am Heart J. 2006;151:713–9.

43. Pisters R, Lane DA, Nieuwlaat R, de Vos CB, Crijns HJ, Lip GY. A novel user- friendly score (HAS-BLED) to assess 1-year risk of major bleeding in patients with atrial fibrillation: the Euro Heart Survey. Chest. 2010;138:1093–100.

44. Fang MC, Go AS, Chang Y, Borowsky LH, Pomernacki NK, Udaltsova N, Singer DE. A new risk scheme to predict warfarin-associated hemorrhage: the ATRIA (Anticoagulation and Risk Factors in Atrial Fibrillation) study. J Am Coll Cardiol. 2011;58:395–401.

45. Hart RG, Pearce LA, Aguilar MI. Meta-analysis: antithrombotic therapy to prevent stroke in patients who have nonvalvular atrial fibrillation. Ann Intern Med. 2007;146:857–67.

46. Odén A, Fahlén M, Hart RG. Optimal INR for prevention of stroke and death in atrial fibrillation: a critical appraisal. Thromb Res. 2006;117(5):493–9.

47. Fang MC, Chang Y, Hylek EM, Rosand J, Greenberg SM, Go AS, Singer DE. Advanced age, anticoagulation intensity, and risk for intracranial hemorrhage among patients taking warfarin for atrial fibrillation. Ann Intern Med. 2004;141(10):745–52.

48. Connolly SJ, Ezekowitz MD, Yusuf S, et al. Dabigatran versus warfarin in patients with atrial fibrillation. N Engl J Med. 2009;361: 1139–51.

49. Patel MR, Mahaffey KW, Garg J, et al. Rivaroxaban versus warfarin in nonvalvular atrial fibrillation. N Engl J Med. 2011;365(10):883–91.

50. Granger CB, Alexander JH, McMurray JJ, et al. Apixaban versus warfarin in patients with atrial fibrillation. N Engl J Med. 2011;365(11):981–92.

51. Banerjee A, Lane DA, Torp-Pedersen C, Lip GY. Net clinical benefit of new oral anticoagulants (dabigatran, rivaroxaban, apixaban) vs. no treatment in a 'real world' atrial fibrillation population: a modelling analysis based on a nationwide cohort study. Thromb Haemost. 2012;107:584–9.

52. Maggioni AD. Acute coronary syndrome in patients with atrial fibrillation. Circulation. 2012;126:1176–8.

53. De Caterina R, Husted S, Wallentin L, Andreotti F, Arnesen H, Bachman F, Baigent C, Hubert K, Jespersen J, Kristensen SD, Lip GYH, Morais J, Rasmussen LH, Siegbahn A, Verheugt FWA, Weitz JI. New oral anticoagulants in atrial fibrillation and acute coronary syndromes. J Am Coll Cardiol. 2012;59:1413–25.

54. Lip GY, Huber K, Andreotti F, Arnesen H, Airaksinen KJ, Cuisset T, Kirchhof P, Marín F. Management of antithrombotic therapy in atrial fibrillation patients presenting with acute coronary syndrome and/or undergoing percutaneous coronary intervention/stenting. Thromb Haemost. 2010;103:13–28.

55. Lamberts M, Olesen JB, Ruwald MH, Hansen CM, Karasoy D, Kristensen SL, Køber L, Torp-Pedersen C, Gislason GH, Hansen ML. Bleeding after initiation of multiple antithrombotic drugs, including triple therapy, in atrial fibrillation patients following myocardial infarction and coronary intervention: a nationwide cohort study. Circulation. 2012;126:1185–93.

56. Sorensen SV, Kansal AR, Connolly S, Peng S, Linnehan J, Bradley-Kennedy C, Plumb JM. Cost-effectiveness of dabigatran etexilate for the prevention of stroke and systemic embolismo in atrial fibrillation: a Canadian payer perspective. Thromb Haemost. 2011;105(5):908–19.

57. Pink J, Lane S, Pirmohamed M, Hughes DA. Dabigatran etexilate versus warfarin in Management of non-valvular atrial fibrillation in UK context: quantitative benefit-harm and economic analyses. BMJ. 2011;343:d6333.

58. Shah SV, Gage BF. Cost-effectiveness of dabigatran for stroke prophylaxis in atrial fibrillation. Circulation. 2011;123(22):2562–70.

59. Freeman JV, Zhu RP, Owens DK, Garber AM, Hutton DW, Go AS, Wang PJ, Turakhia MP. Cost-effectiveness of dabigatran compared with warfarin for stroke prevention in atrial fibrillation. Ann Intern Med. 2011;154(1):1–11.

60. Lee S, Anglade MW, Pisacane R, Kluger J, Coleman CI. Cost-effectiveness of rivaroxaban compared to warfarin for stroke prevention in atrial fibrillation. Am J Cardiol. 2012;110:845–51.

61. González-Juanatey JR, Alvarez-Sabín J, Lobos JM, Martínez-Rubio A, Reverter JC, Oyagüez I, González-Rojas N, Becerra V. Cost-effectiveness of dabigatran for stroke prevention in non-valvular atrial fibrillation in Spain. Rev Esp Cardiol. 2012;65(10):901–10.

Chapter 2
Inside Molecular Mechanisms and Pharmacological Targets of Atrial Fibrillation

Alina Scridon and Dan Dobreanu

Context

Atrial fibrillation (AF) is the most common cardiac arrhythmia, affecting approximately 1 % of the general population and up to 8 % of subjects over the age of 80 years. The presence of the arrhythmia is associated with significant impairment of quality of life, and significant morbidity and mortality from stroke, thromboembolism, and heart failure. According to estimates, the incidence of AF is on increase worldwide and its prevalence is estimated to at least double in the next 50 years.

Growth in the size of the AF population and increased recognition of the morbidity, mortality, and diminished quality of life associated with AF, have spurred numerous investigations to develop more effective therapies for AF and its complications. So far none has provided the expected results. Currently available pharmacological strategies are often inefficient, with enough unpleasant side effects explaining the frequent lack of adherence to treatment. The limited success

A. Scridon, MD, PhD (✉) • D. Dobreanu, MD, PhD
Department of Physiology and Institute of Cardiovascular Disease and Transplant, University of Medicine and Pharmacy of Tîrgu Mures, Tîrgu Mures, Romania
e-mail: alina.scridon@umftgm.ro

G.-A. Dan et al. (eds.), *Atrial Fibrillation Therapy*, Current Cardiovascular Therapy, DOI 10.1007/978-1-4471-5475-4_2, © Springer-Verlag London 2014 in the therapy of AF is highly due to the fact that the precise mechanisms underlying this arrhythmia are poorly understood. It is generally accepted that there is no unifying mechanism of AF, and that one mechanism may predominate over another in certain patients, usually with the participation of several mechanisms in the same patient. A better understanding of the underlying mechanisms is expected to result in more efficient antiarrhythmic strategies and to have a positive impact on the social and economic burdens that AF represents.

Over the past years, much progress has been made in understanding ion channel function, regulation, and remodeling at the molecular level. However, it remains to be established if targeting prevention or reversal of these molecular abnormalities will result in the reduction of the major impact that AF represents and to determine the best time to intervene to lower the risk of occurrence and/or recurrence of atrial arrhythmias.

Pathophysiology of Atrial Fibrillation

Studies performed on animal models identified the classic mechanisms that continue to form the basis for our understanding of the pathophysiology of AF. Two main electrophysiological mechanisms have been proposed in order to explain AF occurrence: focal ectopic activity and reentry circuits, favored by either altered electrical properties or by fixed structural changes of the atrial tissue.

The complex interactions established between these components, which are not mutually exclusive and are likely to co-exist, determine the clinical presentation of the arrhythmia. In the absence of significant substrate, ectopic activity can only induce short, self-terminating episodes of AF (paroxysmal AF), while in the presence of extensively remodeled atria, even limited ectopy can start persistent or permanent AF.

Automatic Focus

Already in the 1940s, Scherf advanced the hypothesis of 'focal AF', based on an animal model in which local administration of aconitine induced focal atrial tachycardia rapidly degenerating into AF [1]. In that model, termination of the arrhythmia could be achieved by isolating the focus of the arrhythmia from the rest of the atrium. Later on, Haïssaguerre et al. identified ectopic activity originating in the pulmonary veins of AF patients [2]. Experiences with AF ablation showed that radiofrequency elimination of pulmonary vein foci could terminate the arrhythmia. However, while pulmonary vein cardiomyocytes probably do contribute to atrial arrhythmias, foci outside the pulmonary veins have also been shown to initiate atrial arrhythmias. Such foci have been described throughout the atria, including the left atrial posterior wall, the right atrium, the superior vena cava, the ligament of Marshall, crista terminalis, and the coronary sinus.

Normal cardiomyocytes present specific electrical activation patterns. Activation of a cardiomyocyte is normally produced by an electrical impulse generated in the sinus node that triggers the opening of the fast Na^+ channels, causing rapid influx of Na^+ ions into the cell. This phase corresponds to the depolarization phase (phase 0 of the action potential), during which the transmembrane potential, initially at a stable resting value of about -80 mV, becomes very positive ($+30$ mV) (Fig. 2.1a). Automatic activity occurs when cardiomyocytes undergo a process of progressive depolarization that interrupts phase 2, phase 3, or phase 4 of the action potential. This phenomenon can occur due to spontaneous diastolic (phase 4) releases of Ca^{2+} from the sarcoplasmic reticulum through ryanodine receptors (RyR) channels, leading to delayed afterdepolarizations (DADs) (Fig. 2.1b), or to a decrease in repolarizing outward K^+ currents, which induce an excessive prolongation of the action potential duration (APD), allowing Ca^{2+} and Na^+ channels to recover their activatability and to create inward Ca^{2+} and/or Na^+ movement

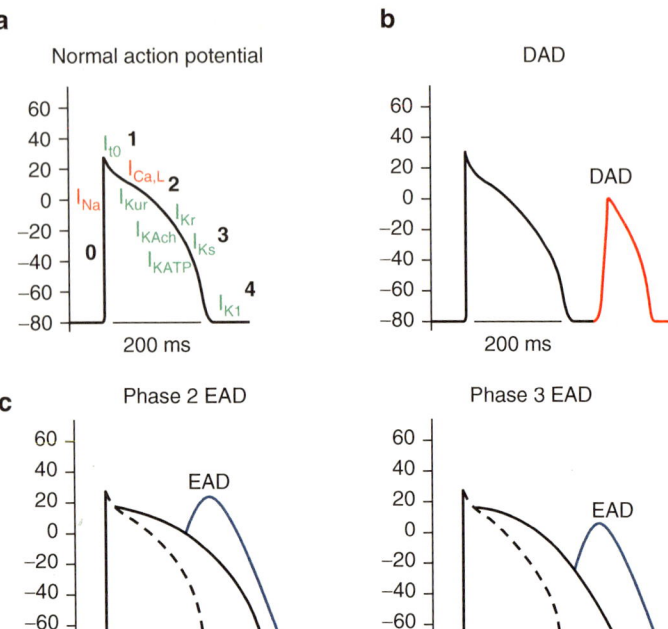

Ion current	Responsible gene
I_{Na}	SCN5A, SCN1B, SCN2B
$I_{Ca,L}$	CACNA1C, CACNB2
I_{t0}	KCND2, KCND3
I_{Kur}	KCNA5
I_{Kr}	KCNH2, KCNE1
I_{Ks}	KCNQ1, KCNE1, KCNE4, KCNE5
I_{KAch}	KCNJ3, KCNJ5
I_{KATP}	ABCC9, KCNJ8, KCNJ11
I_{K1}	KCNJ2, KCNJ4, KCNJ12

FIGURE 2.1 Electrophysiological mechanisms underlying focal ectopic activity. (**a**) Atrial action potential configuration in normal conditions. The five phases of the action potential (*phase 0–4*) and the most relevant inward (*red*) and outward (*green*) ionic currents are depicted. The adjacent panel describes the main genes encoding for each ion current. (**b**) Delayed afterdepolarizations (*DADs*) occur after full repolarization of the cell (*phase 4*) due to spontaneous diastolic releases of Ca^{2+} from the sarcoplasmic reticulum. (**c**) Early afterdepolarizations (*EADs*) occur due to excessive prolongation of the action potential duration, allowing Ca^{2+} and Na^+ channels to recover their activatability and to create inward Ca^{2+} and/or Na^+ movement during action potential phases 2 or 3

---

during action potential phases 2 or 3, leading to early afterdepolarizations (EADs) (Fig. 2.1c). While DADs represent the most important source of ectopic activity in AF, EADs may also be involved in certain cases.

Spontaneous phase 4 releases of Ca^{2+} from the sarcoplasmic reticulum through RyR channels may be due to sarcoplasmic reticulum Ca^{2+} overload, reduced Ca^{2+}-binding to calsequestrin, the main sarcoplasmic reticulum Ca^{2+}-binding protein, or increased sensitivity of RyR channels for Ca^{2+} due to hyperphosphorylation of the channel. Excess intracellular Ca^{2+} then activates the Na^+-Ca^{2+}exchanger, the main mechanism of Ca^{2+} expulsion from the cardiac cell, which will move three ions of Na^+ into the cell for each ion of Ca^{2+} expelled from the cell, generating an inward movement of positive charges and therefore a new depolarization phase (Fig. 2.2).

Reentry Circuits

Reentry defines reexcitation of a myocardial area that has recovered its excitability, by an impulse that previously activated the same region. In AF, reentry can occur due to altered electrical properties or fixed structural changes.

Reentry initiation occurs when a premature ectopic beat, acting as a trigger, encounters refractory tissue when propagating in

FIGURE 2.2 Electrophysiological and molecular mechanisms leading to early (EAD) and delayed (DAD) afterdepolarizations. The most relevant sarcolemmal inward (I_{Na}-sodium current, $I_{Ca,L}$-L-type calcium current) and outward (I_K-rectifier potassium currents) ionic currents and ionic pumps (Na^+/Ca^{2+} exchanger; Na^+/K^+-ATPase) are depicted. Loss of function mutations in KCNA5, the main gene encoding for the ultrarapid delayed rectifier I_{Kur} channel, and missense mutations in the ABCC9 gene, encoding for the ATP-dependent K^+ channel I_{KATP} participate to APD prolongation, allowing Ca^{2+} and Na^+ channels to recover their activatability and to create inward Ca^{2+} and/or Na^+ movement during action potential phases 2 or 3, leading to EADs. Gain of function mutations in the SCN5A gene, encoding for the α-subunit of I_{Na}, could increase the availability of I_{Na} thereby promoting EADs. Ca^{2+} influx through $I_{Ca,L}$ activates ryanodine receptors (RyR) and triggers Ca^{2+} release from the sarcoplasmic reticulum, leading to myocyte contraction. The levels of free cytosolic Ca^{2+} are then regulated by the sarcoplasmic reticulum Ca^{2+}-ATPase ($SERCA$), which refills sarcoplasmic reticulum Ca^{2+} stores after each contraction. The activity of SERCA is regulated by sarcolipin (SLN), a small protein with inhibiting effects on SERCA in association with phospholamban (PLN). The Ca^{2+}-binding protein calsequestrin (CSQ) holds Ca^{2+} inside the sarcoplasmic reticulum after muscle contraction, despite higher concentrations of Ca^{2+} in the sarcoplasmic reticulum than in the cytosol. Spontaneous phase 4 release of Ca^{2+} from the sarcoplasmic reticulum may be due to sarcoplasmic reticulum Ca^{2+} overload, reduced Ca^{2+}-binding to CSQ, or increased sensitivity of RyR channels for Ca^{2+} due to hyperphosphorylation of the channel. Excess intracellular Ca^{2+} then activates the Na^+/Ca^{2+} exchanger, the main mechanism of Ca^{2+} expulsion from the cardiac cell, which will move three ions of Na^+ into the cell for each ion of Ca^{2+} expelled from the cell, generating an inward movement of positive charges and therefore a new depolarization phase. Loss of function mutations and single-nucleotide polymorphisms in the coding region of SLN would promote sarcoplasmic reticulum Ca^{2+} overload due to increased activity of SERCA. Loss of function mutations in the ankyrin (ANK) gene also increase intracellular Ca^{2+} load by reducing the expression of the Na^+/K^+-ATPase and that of the Na^+/Ca^{2+} exchanger, without concomitant changes in Ca^{2+} entry via $I_{Ca,L}$ channels

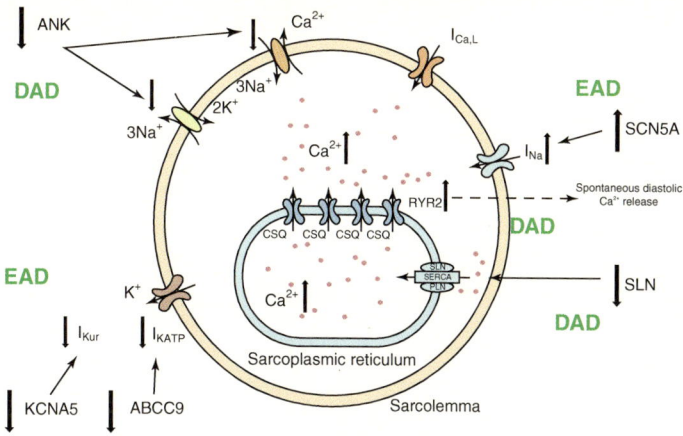

one direction, but it is still able to conduct in the other direction, where the tissue has already recovered, generating a unidirectional block. For the reentry circuit to be maintained, the impulse must cross the circuit slow enough for all points of the circuit to regain their excitability. Thus, the conduction time through the circuit must be longer than its refractory period (Fig. 2.3).

The main determinants of conduction time within the circuit are circuit length and conduction velocity. The longer the circuit length and the slower the velocity of conduction, the more likely is for all points of the circuit to recover their excitability fast enough so that they can be reactivated by the re-circulating impulse. The product between the duration of the refractory period and the velocity of conduction defines the wavelength of the circuit, which determines the size of reentry circuits. Factors that reduce wavelength decrease reentry circuit dimensions, which increase the potential number of simultaneous circuits and augment the probability of AF maintenance.

While structural changes of the atrial myocardium may result in atrial conduction slowing and increased conduction time within the circuit, thus favoring arrhythmia circuits persistence, altered electrical properties of the atrial tissue could result in both atrial conduction slowing, related to changes in sarcolemmal Na^+ channels or gap junctions, and decreased atrial refractoriness due to reduced APD.

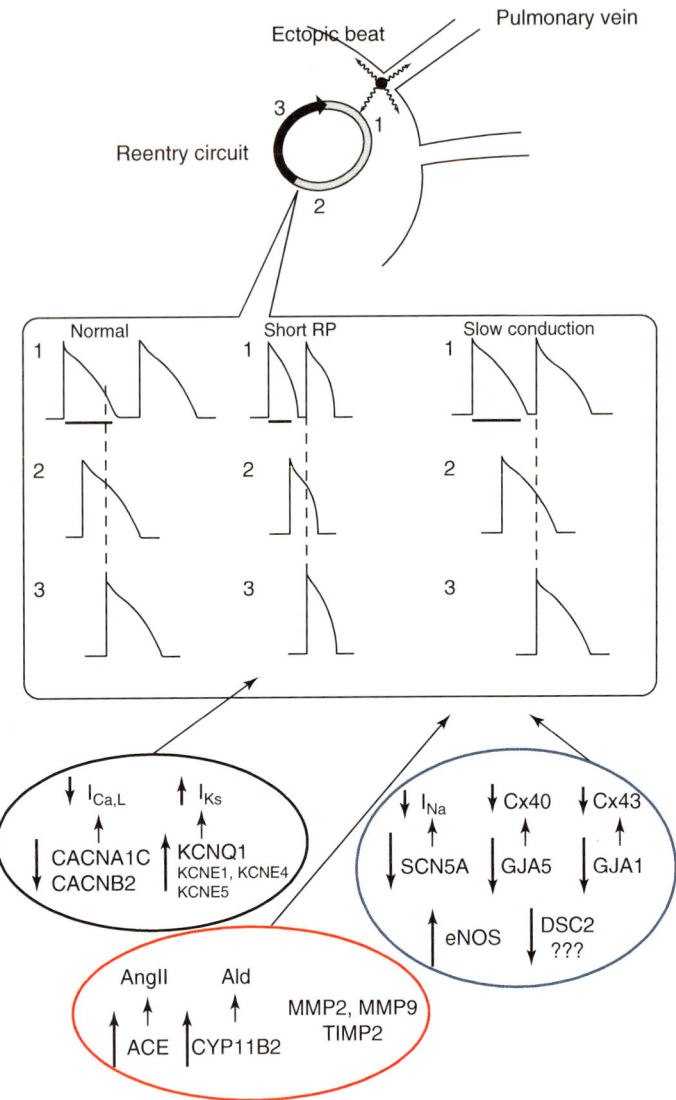

FIGURE 2.3 Electrophysiological and molecular mechanisms leading to reentry. A premature ectopic beat originating in the pulmonary veins blocks in still-refractory cardiac tissue but propagates through excitable tissue (*upper panel*). The *arrow* indicates the leading edge of the wavefront. The *black* area of the *circle* indicates the tissue found in absolute refractory period. The *gray* area of the *circle* indicates the tissue found in relative refractory period. The wavelength of the circuit is defined by the product between the duration of the refractory period (*RP*) and the velocity of conduction. The longer the circuit length and the slower the velocity of conduction, the more likely is for all points of the circuit to recover their excitability fast enough so that they can be reactivated by the re-circulating impulse. The *middle panel* depicts action potentials recorded in different regions of the circuit. In normal conditions (normal atrial refractoriness and conduction) reentry is unlikely to persist (*left*). Shorter APD and refractoriness (*middle*) allows the ectopic beat to reentry the circuit, finding the circuit outside the refractory period. Reduced $I_{Ca,L}$, explaining atrial APD shortening, has been correlated to loss of function mutations in the CACNA1C and CACNB2 genes, encoding for $I_{Ca,L}$ subunits α and β. However, atrial APD shortening is more commonly related to gain of function mutations in genes encoding for outward K^+ currents, such as KCNQ1, KCNE1, KCNE4, or KCNE5, encoding for the slow delayed rectifier I_{Ks}. Conduction slowing maintains the circuit by delaying the arrival of the ectopic impulse until the circuit has regained excitability (*right*). This could be due to molecular mechanisms involved in either alterations in electrical properties (*blue circle*) or structural abnormalities (*red circle*) of the atria. Loss of function mutations in the SCN5A gene, encoding for I_{Na}, promote functional reentry via decreased I_{Na}. Loss of function mutations and polymorphisms in the GJA5 gene, encoding for connexin 40 (*Cx40*), and in the GJA1 gene, encoding for connexin 43 (*Cx43*), impair the intercellular electrical coupling thus slowing the velocity of conduction. Downregulation of the DSC2 gene, encoding for desmocollin 2, might also be related to conduction slowing. Single-nucleotide polymorphisms with gain of function effects in the gene encoding for the endothelial nitric oxide synthase (*eNOS*) might increase the vagal tone and thus decrease atrial conduction velocity. Structural reentry could be favored by polymorphisms with gain of function effects in the angiotensin converting enzyme (*ACE*) gene and in the CYP11B2 gene, encoding for aldosterone synthase, which may affect serum levels of angiotensin II and aldosterone, with pro-fibrotic effects on the myocardium. Several functional polymorphisms in genes encoding for matrix metalloproteinases 2 (*MMP2*) and 9 (*MMP9*), as well as in tissue inhibitor of metalloproteinase 2 (*TIMP2*) also favor arrhythmogenic atrial remodeling

Functional Reentry: Altered Electrical Properties of the Atrial Tissue

The concept of atrial electrical remodeling due to chronic high atrial rates, phenomenon known as 'tachycardia-induced electrical remodeling', was first described in experimental studies [3]. Electrical remodeling primarily occurs due to the very rapid atrial activation and includes changes in ionic properties of atrial myocytes, alterations in sarcolemmal ion channel gene expression, in addition to changes in connexins that couple cells electrically. Action potential recordings and patch clamp experiments in isolated atrial cells from animal models and patients with chronic AF showed a consistent pattern. Reduced APD and refractoriness, together with the loss of physiological rate-adaptation of APD, are the most common electrical changes encountered in this setting.

These abnormalities are probably largely due to impaired Ca^{2+} homeostasis. A significant 63 % reduction in the density of L-type calcium current ($I_{Ca,L}$) was observed in atrial myocytes of patients with chronic AF [4]. Increased atrial rate in these patients induces Ca^{2+} overload in atrial myocytes. Given that Ca^{2+} overload exhibits cytotoxic effects on cardiac cells, decreased $I_{Ca,L}$ could then occur as an adaptive, protective mechanism. Decreased $I_{Ca,L}$ would decrease indeed Ca^{2+} loading of atrial cells, but would simultaneously lead to shortening of the APD, shortening atrial refractory periods and decreasing the wavelength, thus favoring multiple reentry circuits and perpetuation of the arrhythmia. Increased inward repolarizing rectifier K^+ current I_{K1} and constitutively active acetylcholine-dependent current (I_{KAch}), have also been incriminated in APD shortening in this context [5]. Furthermore, increased inward K^+ currents could also favor the arrhythmia by hyperpolarizing atrial cells and triggering afterdepolarizations [6].

A significant reduction in sodium currents (I_{Na}) density was also reported in the presence of AF [7]. While the decrease in $I_{Ca,L}$ leads to a reduction in APD, the reduction in I_{Na} could contribute to the decrease in conduction velocity. These changes concurrently facilitate reentry mechanisms. In various studies, the transient outward potassium current (I_{to}) and the ultrarapid delayed rectifier potassium current (I_{Kur}) were also found to be reduced [8].

Anatomical Reentry: Fixed Structural Changes

The extracellular matrix provides the skeleton for cardiomyocyte alignment, the basis for force transmission, and assures the geometry of the atria. Substantial changes in the composition of the extracellular matrix, such as abnormal collagen deposition and fibrosis within the atrial tissue impair atrial conductibility, increase the heterogeneity of atrial conduction, thus providing a structural basis for reentry. Experimental studies demonstrated that structural abnormalities often precede the onset of AF, since they emanate from senescence, cardiac damage due to coronary artery disease, hemodynamic overload from valve disease or hypertension. Structural alterations comprise a wide range of cellular and ultrastructural abnormalities, with components varying depending particularly on coexisting cardiac conditions and specie.

Regardless of the model, a consistent finding is that of the major heterogeneity of lesions, not only within different sites, but also regionally, with severely injured myocytes next to virtually unaltered cells. However, structural lesions observed in humans with AF seem to be more severe and more extensive than those observed in animal models of AF. The presence of concomitant heart conditions could be at least partially responsible for these findings.

Molecular Mechanisms of Atrial Fibrillation

Molecular research in AF has focused on two main fields: identification of genes involved in AF occurrence and identification of altered gene expression during AF.

Possible genes responsible for AF onset include genes that affect automaticity, atrial refractory period duration and conduction. However, resequencing of AF patient cohorts suggests that recognized mutations account for only a small fraction of all AF cases, and that familial forms of AF are quite uncommon. Most of the remaining cases represent acquired forms of AF and can be related to various structural abnormalities. However, not all individuals presenting cardiac pathologies develop AF. This observation suggests that genetic factors might also contribute to AF propensity in certain patients. Association studies showed that common genetic variants, single-nucleotide polymorphisms, are much more frequent, though they act with a weaker effect and a less-clear phenotype.

Studies designed to assess altered gene expression mainly provide insights into the molecular changes induced by the presence of the arrhythmia itself. It remains to be established if these molecular abnormalities actually participate to the etiology of the arrhythmia, or if they represent an epiphenomenon.

Genetic Bases of Focal Ectopic Activity

Several gene mutations and single-nucleotide polymorphisms have been associated with increased atrial automaticity, generally due to altered ion channels function (Fig. 2.2).

Although Ca^{2+}-handling is considered a culprit feature in the pathophysiology of AF, only a small number of studies reported an implication of gene mutations involving Ca^{2+} pathways in the onset of AF. Several mutations and loss of function single-nucleotide polymorphisms in the coding region of sarcolipin (SLN), a small protein of the membrane of the sarcoplasmic reticulum, possessing an inhibiting effect on Ca^{2+} pumps of cardiac and skeletal muscles in association with phospholamban, have been associated with AF [9]. Loss of function mutations in the ankyrin (ANK) gene have also been incriminated in AF occurrence [10]. Mutations in this gene impair intracellular Ca^{2+}-handling by reducing the expression of the Na^+/K^+-ATPase and that of the Na^+/Ca^{2+} exchanger, without concomitant changes in Ca^{2+} entry via $I_{Ca,L}$ channels. Increased intracellular Ca^{2+} levels could then favor early and delayed afterdepolarizations, which in turn could trigger AF.

Loss of function mutations in KCNA5, the main gene encoding for the ultra rapid delayed rectifier I_{Kur} channel, have also been associated with AF [11]. This is quite surprising, given that decreased I_{Kur} would be expected to prolong APD and atrial refractoriness. However, deficit in KCNA5 expression seems to increase susceptibility to arrhythmogenic EADs and stress-induced atrial arrhythmias [12].

Gain of function mutations associated with AF also involve the SCN5A gene, encoding for the α-subunit of the cardiac Na^+ channel [13]. However, to date, the extent to which SCN5A mutations are related with AF remains unclear. These mutations could increase Na^+ channel availability, promoting atrial ectopic activity.

Additionally, missense mutations in the ABCC9 gene, encoding for the ATP-dependent K^+ channel I_{KATP}, appear to confer an increased susceptibility to adrenergic AF originating in the vein of Marshall [14].

Genetic Bases of Functional Reentry

Molecular abnormalities leading to functional reentry include both gene mutations and single-nucleotide polymorphisms responsible of APD shortening and conduction slowing (Fig. 2.3). These abnormalities include loss of function mutations in genes encoding for various subunits of $I_{Ca,L}$ channels, gain of function mutations in genes encoding for K^+ channels, as well as loss of function mutations in genes encoding for proteins that exhibit gap junction activity.

Reduced $I_{Ca,L}$, explaining atrial APD shortening, has been correlated to loss of function mutations in the CACNA1C and CACNB2 genes, encoding for $I_{Ca,L}$ subunits α and β, in a cohort of patients with Brugada syndrome or short-QT electrocardiographic phenotypes who also presented AF [15].

However, atrial APD shortening is more commonly related to gain of function mutations in genes encoding for outward

K⁺ currents, including KCNQ1, KCNE2, KCNH2, and KCNJ2 [16–18]. A missense mutation in the KCNQ1 gene, encoding for the α-subunit of the slow delayed rectifier I_{Ks} current was the first gene mutation associated with AF [16]. The mutation was identified in a four-generation Chinese family with autosomal dominantly inherited lone AF. Functional studies confirmed a gain of function in I_{Ks}, explaining the shortening of atrial APD and refractoriness. Other mutations have been identified in several of the regulating subunits of I_{Ks}. A mutation in the KCNE2 gene was identified in two Chinese families with lone AF [19]. Functional analyses revealed a gain of function effect in I_{Ks} leading to a shortening of the APD. Single-nucleotide polymorphisms in the KCNE1, KCNE4 and KCNE5 genes, leading to gain of function effects on I_{Ks}, have also been associated with an increased propensity to AF [20–22]. Furthermore, given that KCNE5 is located on chromosome X, this finding could also help to explain the higher risk of AF in men. However, it remains to be established how certain gain of function mutations in outward K⁺ channels manage to induce shortening of the APD at the atrial level, while leaving ventricular repolarization unaltered or even prolonging it.

Several other mutations promote AF by targeting ion channels or membrane proteins that govern conduction velocity, inducing conduction slowing.

Of particular interest are mutations in SCN5A. While gain of function mutations in this gene promote ectopic activity within the atria [13], as previously discussed, loss of function mutations in the same gene could promote functional reentry, via decreased I_{Na} and conduction slowing [23]. Additionally, two single-nucleotide polymorphisms in the SCN1B gene and two in the SCN2B gene were also identified in AF populations, also leading to a loss of function effect in I_{Na} [24].

Experimental data suggested that nitric oxide participates to vagal cardiac activity, while inhibiting adrenergic activity. The significant association between AF and certain single-nucleotide polymorphisms with gain of function effects in the gene encoding for the endothelial nitric oxide synthase (eNOS) suggests a participation of eNOS in atrial arrhythmogenicity related to an increased vagal tone and decreased atrial conduction velocity [25].

Accumulating data suggest a close association between abnormal expression of genes encoding for proteins that exhibit gap junction activity and AF. The GJA5 gene encodes for connexin-40, which is particularly important in the atria. In a report by Hagendorff et al., the authors subjected connexin-40 heterozygous and homozygous knockout mice to rapid atrial transesophageal stimulation [26]. In mice that were either connexin-40 intact or heterozygous there was no evidence of inducible arrhythmias. In contrast, in connexin-40 deficient mice burst pacing generated atrial arrhythmias in 63 % of animals. Both GJA5 mutations and polymorphisms have been observed in AF patients [27]. In patients with rheumatic heart disease, reduction and redistribution of connexins-43, encoded by the GJA1 gene, was also shown to contribute to both initiation and persistence of AF [28]. Recent data suggest that downregulation of the DSC2 gene, encoding for desmocollin 2, might also be related to AF (unpublished data). Mutations in this gene are known to cause arrhythmogenic right ventricular cardiomyopathy, an inherited channelopathy associated with increased risk of ventricular arrhythmias. Several clinical studies reported increased incidence of supraventricular arrhythmias in patients with arrhythmogenic right ventricular cardiomyopathy and high prevalence of sustained AF induced at electrophysiological study compared to patients without cardiac disease. Although the precise mechanisms that underlie this predisposition are not entirely known, DSC2 downregulation in atrial myocytes could provide an answer.

Genetic Bases of Structural Reentry

Studies performed on animal models emphasized conduction abnormalities favoring unidirectional conduction block and reentry, conduction heterogeneities secondary to regional fibrotic differences, and focal atrial activity, as potential mechanisms for atrial fibrosis-related arrhythmias. However, pathophysiological and genetic factors that promote atrial fibrosis remain incompletely understood (Fig. 2.3).

Genetic polymorphisms within various genes of the renin-angiotensin system have been associated with non-familial AF. Insertion/deletion polymorphisms in the angiotensin converting enzyme (ACE) gene have been identified in several large studies. These polymorphisms may affect serum levels of angiotensin II, known for its pro-fibrotic effects on the myocardium. The presence of a D allele in the ACE gene was associated with decreased breakdown of type I collagen, while treatment with ACE inhibitors has been shown to increase type I collagen breakdown [29]. Additionally, it appears that angiotensin II also augments $I_{Ca,L}$ and trans-membrane Ca^{2+} movements. Increased transmembrane Ca^{2+} movements could then initiate late phase 3 EADs, an important mechanism of rapid firing within the pulmonary veins. Furthermore, increased $I_{Ca,L}$ could induce spatial dispersion of repolarization within the atrium, generating conduction block, reentry, and initiation of AF. Various polymorphisms in the CYP11B2 gene, encoding for aldosterone synthase, have also been associated with atrial structural remodeling and AF occurrence [30]. A significant association was also observed between AF and a polymorphism in the AGT gene, encoding for angiotensinogen, in a Chinese population [31].

Matrix metalloproteinases (MMPs) have been associated with arrhythmogenic atrial remodeling and with the persistence of AF. Several functional MMP9 polymorphisms, leading to an altered expression of MMP9 proteins, can modulate the susceptibility to AF [32]. MMP2 and its inhibitor, TIMP2, also play an important role in the pathophysiology of arrhythmogenic atrial remodeling and can contribute to AF occurrence and persistence [33].

PITX2: The Panaceas of Atrial Fibrillation

Genome-wide association studies identified three genetic loci on chromosomes 4q25, 16q22, and 1q21 associated with AF [34, 35]. The single-nucleotide polymorphisms most significantly associated with AF are located on chromosome 4q25, in a 'genomic desert' – a large, intergenic region, without any known genes. The closest gene in the region is PITX2, a member of the pituitary homeobox family of transcription factors that plays an important role in early morphogenesis, being responsible of the left-right asymmetry of the heart, and differentially regulating left atrial identity and ventricular asymmetrical remodeling programs. PITX2 also plays essential roles in regulating the development of cardiac conduction system, particularly the sinus node, but also that of the left atrium and the pulmonary vein myocardium.

Chinchilla et al. were the first to demonstrate that PITX2 is significantly decreased in patients with sustained AF, providing a molecular link between PITX2 loss of function and AF [36]. However, it seems that PITX2 expression is not altered in the developmental period, but its impairment only occurs in the adult heart. Reports in PITX2$^{-/-}$ knockout mice showed that these animals present right atrial isomerism and both atrial and ventricular septal defects and die before birth [37]. Thus, it is more likely for a dysfunction acquired in adulthood to underlie PITX2 downregulation-related predisposition to AF.

Although the involvement of PITX2 in AF occurrence has been extensively studied in the last years, pathophysiological pathways that relate PITX2 loss of function to AF remain incompletely understood. Accumulating data indicate that PITX2 might play a role in atrial automaticity, as well as in functional and anatomical reentry.

PITX2 Involvement in Focal Ectopic Activity

All cardiomyocytes of the developing heart initially possess pacemaker properties, but only a small proportion of cells differentiate into pacemaker cells and PITX2 plays a crucial role in this process. PITX2 represses SHOX2, a transcription factor expressed in sinus node precursors. Repression of SHOX2 by PITX2 results in downregulation of a nodal gene program and upregulation of a gene program characteristic for a working myocardium phenotype. Because PITX2 expression is restricted to left atrial SHOX2 expression, the development of the sinus node is only repressed in the left atrium. In the right atrium, missing PITX2 will result in SHOX2 upregulation. Consequently, certain cardiomyocytes of the right atrium will express a nodal gene program, and eventually create the sinus node. PITX2 downregulation in left atrial cardiomyocytes observed in AF patients could thus participate to the increased left atrial arrhythmogenicity in this population [38].

Additionally, PITX2 loss of function has also been associated with a slight overexpression in the HCN4 gene, encoding for the pacemaker current I_f [38]. Given that PITX2 is essential for the development of pulmonary veins, PITX2 loss of function could also be involved in the automatic activity of pulmonary veins.

PITX2 Involvement in Functional Reentry

PITX2 seems to modulate the expression of various ion channels, and therein provide molecular substrates for atrial arrhythmogenesis. In a study of Kirchoff et al., PITX2$^{-/+}$ hearts were susceptible to AF elicited by programmed stimulation with a single atrial premature beat [39]. The authors also showed that reduced expression of PITX2 in these mice caused shortening of atrial APD. Gene expression patterns and functional analyses in PITX2 deficient atria indicated that modified Ca^{2+}-handling, cell-cell communication, or altered function of melanocytes could participate to AF predisposition in this setting.

Microarray analysis of mutant PITX2 null mice showed overexpression of several genes encoding for K^+ channels, including KCNQ1 (encoding for the α-subunit of I_{Ks}) and KNCK2 (encoding for a stretch-activated K^+ channel), which could again explain APD shortening in this setting as well as the propensity of these animals to AF.

In addition, PITX2 misexpression has been shown to impair connexin-40 expression, both in embryonic stem cell-derived cardiomyocytes and in fetal and adult atrial and ventricular chamber-specific PITX2 loss of function mice [40]. These data provide a putative link to AF, since mutations in connexin-40 gene are associated with AF and further implicate impaired PITX2 function at adult stages in predisposition to AF.

PITX2 Involvement in Structural Reentry

The fact that PITX2 is a transcription factor that regulates the genetic expression of procollagen lysyl hydroxylase, an enzyme mandatory for collagen formation and stabilization, suggests a potential participation of PITX2 in LA structural remodeling [41].

However, it remains unclear whether AF triggers PITX2 downregulation or whether the presence of pre-existing PITX2 downregulation promotes AF. Further studies will have to provide an answer.

Altered Gene Expression During Atrial Fibrillation

With the exception of relatively rare cases of lone AF, in which genetic factors seem to play a culprit role, the arrhythmia is commonly associated with various other cardiac conditions. In fact, an underlying heart disease is present in 70 % of patients with AF. The presence of these comorbidities creates a substrate for acquired forms of AF and complicates therapy for these patients.

The presence of these comorbidities induces characteristic gene expression changes within the atria. Genes generally express their function by the means of a protein. The two main steps in the transition from a gene to the resulting protein are transcription and translation. Under the influence of appropriate stimuli, a first phase of transcription is triggered inside the nucleus. Messenger ribonucleic acids (mRNAs) are thus produced from the deoxyribonucleic acid sequence of the gene. The totality of mRNAs present in a cell at a given time defines the transcriptome of that cell. Unlike for the genome, the 'composition' of the transcriptome is constantly changing as a result of newly generated mRNAs and enzymatic degradation of other mRNAs. The transcriptome is a highly dynamic structure that reflects cell's adaptation to its environment. In AF patients, transcriptome analysis showed a consistent pattern of expression changes, including alterations in genes encoding for ion channels and Ca^{2+}-handling proteins, oxidative stress, and a ventricular-like expression signature [42]. However, the exact molecular mechanisms involved in these adaptation processes during AF are far from clear. Identification of the signaling pathways and their target genes could lead to new therapeutic options for AF patients.

While some of these molecular changes seem to be related to the presence of AF itself as part of the AF-induced left atrial electrical and structural remodeling, others could emanate from coexisting cardiac conditions.

Pathophysiological Mechanisms Promoting Atrial Fibrillation

Concomitant pathophysiological processes, such as autonomic imbalance, inflammation, oxidative stress, or various changes in the renin-angiotensin system, are known to trigger and/or aggravate one or several of the electrophysiological mechanisms underlying AF. At their turn, these pathophysiological processes are generally the result of coexisting conditions, such as arterial hypertension, heart failure, myocardial infarction, diabetes, or obesity, explaining the high incidence of AF in these settings (Fig. 2.4).

Sympatho-vagal imbalance is largely accepted as a main trigger for AF onset. However, while electrical and structural remodeling are recognized as key pieces in the vicious circle by which AF favors AF, recent data suggest that autonomic remodeling also participates to the auto-perpetuation of AF. It seems that during AF, increased cardiac filling pressure and

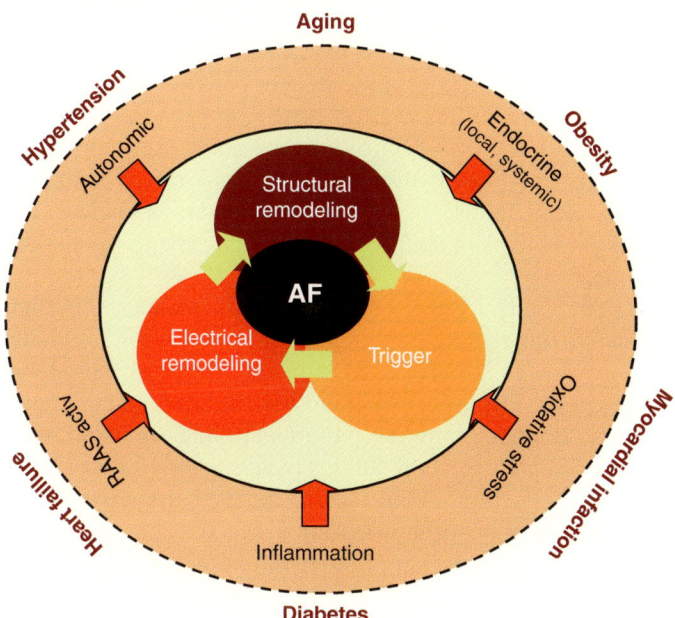

FIGURE 2.4 Schematic representation of the relationship between electrophysiological mechanisms underlying atrial fibrillation (*AF*; *inner circles*), pathophysiological mechanisms promoting AF (*middle circle*), and cardiac and non-cardiac conditions triggering these later pathophysiological mechanisms (*outer circle*). *RAAS* renin-angiotensin-aldosteron system

decreased arterial blood pressure send conflicting messages, confusing the autonomic nervous system [43]. While the decreased cardiac output leads to unloading of arterial baro-receptors and reflex sympatho-excitation, the increase in fill-ing pressure leads to activation of cardiopulmonary baroreceptors and sympatho-inhibition. The importance of each of these mechanisms seems to vary from one individual to another. Impaired autonomic function induced by the presence of AF could then further favor the persistence of the arrhythmia, mainly by altering ion channels function. While increased vagal tone shortens the effective refractory period and increases the dispersion of refractoriness, leading to an increased number of functional obstacles and hence wavebreaks and generating new wavelets, heterogeneous sympathetic hyperinnervation of the atria could lead to an increase in the dispersion of refractoriness. Autonomic dysfunctions have been observed in various other conditions, such as heart failure, myocardial infarction, or diabetes, and could partly explain the propensity of the arrhythmia in these settings.

Both clinical and experimental studies highlight *inflammation* as a modulating factor predisposing to AF, due to a process of inflammation-induced structural remodeling and fibrosis. The exact mechanisms that link inflammation to tissue remodeling in AF patients are unclear and deserve further research. Several studies have suggested that inflammation exerts remodeling effects through *reactive oxygen species*. It has been shown that C-reactive protein (CRP) promotes the generation of reactive oxygen species by altering the homeostatic balance of pro-oxidants-antioxidative enzymes in endothelial progenitor cells. Oxygen-free radicals can also activate MMPs generating an imbalance between accumulation and breakdown of extracellular matrix, thus enhancing LA fibrosis. Alternatively, rapid atrial activation could lead to intracellular accumulation of Ca^{2+} within atrial myocytes and in some cases to initiation of apoptotic loss of atrial myocytes. CRP might then bind to the damaged atrial myocytes, inducing a local low-grade inflammatory response, and consequent fibrosis. Moreover, phosphatidylcholine degradation that occurs during this process could also inhibit the exchange of Na^+ and Ca^{2+} ions in sarcomeres, further promoting AF maintenance. Inflammation probably plays crucial roles in settings such as postoperative AF. AF has been shown to occur in up to 40 % of patients undergoing cardiac bypass surgery and in up to 50 % of patients undergoing cardiac valvular surgery. The inflammatory cascade and catecholamine surge associated with surgery are thought to play the prominent role in AF initiation in this setting. In post-cardiac surgery patients, CRP levels peak on post-operative day 2, with complement-CRP complexes peaking on post-operative day 2 or 3, whereas the incidence of AF follows a similar pattern and peaks on post-operative day 2 or 3. However, in the majority of clinical settings, it remains unclear whether initiation of AF activates inflammatory pathways or whether the presence of a pre-existing systemic inflammatory status promotes further persistence of AF.

It is largely accepted that hyperactivation of the **renin-angiotensin system** participates to the pathogenesis of AF through numerous mechanisms, including left atrial structural remodeling and fibrosis, modulation of ion channels and gap junctions, as well as increased ectopic activity within the pulmonary veins. Renin-angiotensin system hyperactivity is one of the main pathways responsible of interstitial atrial fibrosis and consequently conduction slowing and heterogeneity, and this is mainly due to the pro-inflammatory and pro-fibrotic effects of angiotensin II. Angiotensin II triggers an alteration in extracellular matrix composition by directly promoting fibroblast proliferation and collagen synthesis, resulting in excessive collagen deposition, but also by diminishing collagen degradation due to MMPs and TIMP concentrations imbalance [44]. Furthermore, angiotensin II has been shown to downregulate I_{to}, favoring reentry, but can also induce DADs and accelerate automatic rhythm within pulmonary vein cardiomyocytes. Angiotensin II could also exert proarrhythmic effects by impairing gap junctions, such as connexin-43 [45].

The extent to which the pathophysiological mechanisms of AF participate to arrhythmia occurrence is largely dependent on the underlying cardiac condition.

In experimental models of heart failure induced by right ventricular tachypacing, structural remodeling seems to play the major role in AF occurrence. Atrial effective refractory period appears to be unchanged or increased by congestive heart failure, but localized regions of conduction slowing occur in association with marked atrial fibrosis. Cessation of ventricular tachypacing allowed ventricular function and atrial dilation to reverse completely, along with the disappearance of hemodynamic and clinical signs of congestive heart failure, but fibrosis remained and the ability to induce prolonged AF was maintained [46].

Several of the pathological mechanisms previously mentioned are strongly influenced by aging. Senescence is not only accompanied by an important process of cardiac fibrosis, but also induces significant morphological changes in the action potential, including a decrease in peak and plateau action potential voltage, a decrease in the rate of cellular depolarization, a slight decrease in resting membrane potential, and an increased dispersion of APD across the tissue [47]. Thus, fibrosis, slowed conduction of premature beats, and increased heterogeneity of repolarization could be important determinants of both initiation and maintenance of AF in the elderly.

In various experimental models of arterial hypertension, widespread conduction abnormalities and atrial wavelength shortening could be observed [48]. However, refractoriness does not seem to change significantly. Atrial tissue presents significant structural remodeling, including central myofibrillolysis, myocyte hypertrophy, mitochondrial and nuclear enlargement and fibrosis, as well as evidence of apoptosis. Furthermore, the presence of arterial hypertension seems to accelerate the remodeling process induced by aging, probably due to a combination of factors such as earlier development and more severe diastolic dysfunction, impaired plasma volume control, intensified neurohormonal activation, and atrial myopathy secondary to oxidative stress and lipoapoptosis.

Obesity is also associated with a 0.5-fold higher risk of AF in both men and women, probably mediated by complex mechanisms involving LA structural remodeling, increased production of pro-inflammatory proteins, neurally mediated mechanisms with vagal modulation of atrial electrophysiology through fat pads, or endothelial dysfunction mediated through a paracrine mechanism [49].

Molecular Targets in Atrial Fibrillation

The increasing incidence of AF imposes more effective therapies for AF and its complications. Currently available antiarrhythmic agents, that usually block voltage-gated ion channels, are often inefficient and are frequently associated with disconcerting side-effects. The increasing number of experimental studies in clinically relevant pathological substrates for AF provided new insights into the pathophysiological mechanisms of the arrhythmia. Consequently, new therapeutic strategies have emerged, and 'upstream therapy' of AF, a mechanism-based approach, was expected to provide promising results. Experimental use of various agents targeting the renin-angiotensin system, inflammation, or oxidative stress demonstrated indeed beneficial effects of these agents on AF prophylaxis and/or treatment.

Recognition of the participation of the renin-angiotensin system in AF occurrence has spurred numerous studies to assess the efficacy of ACE inhibitors, antialdosteronics, or angiotensin II receptor blockers in AF prevention and/or treatment. While increased angiotensin II production in transgenic mice with cardiac-restricted ACE overexpression caused marked atrial dilation, focal fibrosis and AF [50], both AF susceptibility and atrial fibrosis could be decreased by candesartan or enalapril, but not by hydralazine or isosorbid mononitrate, despite similar hemodynamic effects [51, 52]. These results indicated a potent antiarrhythmic effect of renin-angiotensin system blockade, which is not limited to improved hemodynamics. A meta-analysis of all trials using ACE inhibitors and angiotensin II receptor blockers showed that these drugs possess indeed quite potent antiarrhythmic effects [53]. In the overall population, these drugs reduced new-onset AF by 18 %, and among heart failure patients as much as 43 %. Statins have also shown a benefit for the primary prevention of AF, but they were less efficient for preventing AF recurrences after cardioversion or ablation [54]. Despite the fact that *omega*-3-acid ethyl esters are thought to exhibit antiarrhythmic effects by attenuating the inflammatory status, the endothelial dysfunction, the oxidative stress, and stabilizing cell membrane, currently available data regarding *omega*-3-acid ethyl esters efficacy in AF prevention or treatment are scarce and contradictory [55]. Therefore, the efficacy of the majority of these mechanism-based strategies remains questionable and is probably largely dependent on the substrate of the arrhythmia and coexisting cardiac conditions. Moreover, it remains to be established the best time to intervene.

Recent studies assessing the molecular mechanisms linked to AF allowed further insights into understanding ion channel function, regulation, and remodeling and provided new therapeutic targets. However, it remains to be established if targeting prevention or reversal of these molecular abnormalities will result in reduction of the major impact that AF represents and to determine the best time to intervene to lower the risk of occurrence and/or recurrence of atrial arrhythmias.

Given that ectopic automatic activity usually results from spontaneous diastolic releases of Ca^{2+} from the sarcoplasmic reticulum through RyR2 channels, sarcoplasmic reticulum dysfunction prevention by RyR2 stabilizing agents could offer promising results. A new experimental drug, JTV-519 (K201), a 1,4-benzothiazepine analogue, originally discovered due to its cardioprotective effects in a model of myocardial injury, appears to block intracellular Ca^{2+} overload by nonspecifically inhibiting Na^+, Ca^{2+}, and K^+ currents [56]. Additionally, JTV-519 could exert therapeutic effects due to a stabilizing effect on the interaction between RyR2 and calstabin2, a Ca^{2+} channel-stabilizing binding protein [57]. RyR2 blocking agents, such as the local anesthetic drug tetracaine or the class IC antiarrhythmic agent flecainide, could also be of therapeutic value [58]. Both of these agents prevent DADs by effectively inhibiting Ca^{2+} leaks from the sarcoplasmic reticulum. Additionally, Ca^{2+} leaks from the sarcoplasmic reticulum could also be reduced by blocking Ca^{2+}/calmodulin-dependent protein kinase hyperphosphorylation of RyR2, either directly or indirectly by inhibition of calmodulin [59]. Attempts to use Ca^{2+} channel blockers to treat AF showed no benefit on atrial remodeling, despite the fact that, at least in theory, they should reduce Ca^{2+} overload [60]. However, given that decreased $I_{Ca,L}$ is a key contributor to AF occurrence, Ca^{2+} channel blockade could in fact promote AF persistence [61]. Upstream strategies, designed to prevent $I_{Ca,L}$ downregulation might offer new therapeutic insights.

Recognition of APD shortening as a key step in AF occurrence and maintenance suggested class III, APD-prolonging, arrhythmic agents as potentially beneficial drugs. However, their effect on I_{Kr} and the increased risk of malignant ventricular arrhythmias due to EADs limits their use. This inconvenience could be overcome by targeting atrial-specific ion channels, while avoiding the deleterious effects on ventricular repolarization phase. One new antiarrhythmic agent, vernakalant, appears to be efficient and safe for conversion of short-duration AF to sinus rhythm [62]. This drug is a relatively atrial-selective compound, blocking early-activating potassium currents and frequency-dependent sodium current, while not significantly affecting the length of the QT interval. Targeting I_{Kur} or I_{KAch} channels, which are well expressed in the atria, but absent in the ventricles, could represent other therapeutic approaches. However, it appears that I_{Kur} blockade might predispose to repolarization-related arrhythmias in adrenergic settings [11].

Dysfunction of proteins involved in intercellular communication may be important in the maintenance of AF. Thus, ameliorating connexin function might represent a promising new therapeutic strategy. Antiarrhythmic peptides such as rotigaptide proved to be effective against mitral regurgitation or acute ischemia-related AF, but not in the context of heart failure [63]. These discordant findings are probably due to different participation of connexin dysfunction in arrhythmia onset, according to the substrate of the arrhythmia.

Accumulating data suggest that the PITX2 downregulation-AF relationship is very important. Therefore, it would seem reasonable to hypothesize that timely appropriate therapy designed to block PITX2 downregulation in these patients might prevent and/or treat AF. However, to date, no study has identified the mechanisms responsible of PITX2 insufficiency in AF patients.

Beside the potential use of these molecular mechanisms as therapeutic targets, genetic studies could also help identify patients who will benefit most from various therapeutic strategies, or, contrarily, who would be at high risk of proarrhythmia if treated with channel-blocking agents. It is also crucial to remember that AF is a very complex disease, and that the phenotype of the arrhythmia probably results from a complex assembling of genetic defects and environmental factors. Therefore, targeting a unique mechanism of the arrhythmia cannot be expected to provide impressing results.

References

1. Scherf D. Studies on auricular tachycardia caused by aconitine administration. Proc Soc Exp Biol Med. 1947;4:233–9.
2. Haïssaguerre M, Marcus FI, Fischer B, et al. Radiofrequency catheter ablation in unusual mechanisms of atrial fibrillation: report of three cases. J Cardiovasc Electrophysiol. 1994;5:743–51.
3. Wijffels MC, Kirchhof CJ, Dorland R, et al. Atrial fibrillation begets atrial fibrillation. A study in awake chronically instrumented goats. Circulation. 1995;92:1954–68.
4. Van Wagoner DR, Pond AL, Lamorgese M, et al. Atrial L-Type Ca2+ currents and human atrial fibrillation. Circ Res. 1999;85:428–36.
5. Ehrlich JR. Inward rectifier potassium currents as a target for atrial fibrillation therapy. J Cardiovasc Pharmacol. 2008;52(2):129–35.
6. Cha TJ, Ehrlich JR, Zhang L, et al. Atrial tachycardia remodeling of pulmonary vein cardiomyocytes: comparison with left atrium and potential relation to arrhythmogenesis. Circulation. 2005;111(6):728–35.
7. Gaspo R, Bosch RF, Bou-Abboud E, et al. Tachycardia-induced changes in Na+ current in a chronic dog model of atrial fibrillation. Circ Res. 1997;81:1045–52.
8. Bosch RF, Zeng X, Grammer JB, et al. Ionic mechanisms of electrical remodeling in human atrial fibrillation. Cardiovasc Res. 1999;44:121–31.
9. Nyberg MT, Stoevring B, Behr ER, et al. The variation of the sarcolipin gene (SLN) in atrial fibrillation, long QT syndrome and sudden arrhythmic death syndrome. Clin Chim Acta. 2007;375:87–91.
10. Mohler PJ, Schott JJ, Gramolini AO, et al. Ankyrin-B mutation causes type 4 long-QT cardiac arrhythmia and sudden cardiac death. Nature. 2003;421(6923):634–9.
11. Olson TM, Alekseev AE, Liu XK, et al. Kv1.5 channelopathy due to KCNA5 loss-of-function mutation causes human atrial fibrillation. Hum Mol Genet. 2006;15(14):2185–91.

12. Feng J, Wible B, Li G, et al. Antisense oligodeoxynucleotides directed against Kv1.5 mRNA specifically inhibit ultrarapid delayed rectifier K+current in cultured adult human atrial myocytes. Circ Res. 1997;80:572–9.
13. Makiyama T, Akao M, Shizuta S, et al. A novel SCN5A gain-of-function mutation M1875T associated with familial atrial fibrillation. J Am Coll Cardiol. 2008;52(16):1326–34.
14. Olson TM, Alekseev AE, Moreau C, et al. KATP channel mutation confers risk for vein of Marshall adrenergic atrial fibrillation. Nat Clin Pract Cardiovasc Med. 2007;4(2):110–6.
15. Antzelevitch C, Pollevick GD, Cordeiro JM, et al. Loss-of-function mutations in the cardiac calcium channel underlie a new clinical entity characterized by ST-segment elevation, short QT intervals, and sudden cardiac death. Circulation. 2007;115(4):442–9.
16. Chen YH, Xu SJ, Bendahhou S, et al. KCNQ1 gain-of-function mutation in familial atrial fibrillation. Science. 2003;299(5604): 251–4.
17. Tsai CT, Lai LP, Hwang JJ, et al. Molecular genetics of atrial fibrillation. J Am Coll Cardiol. 2008;52(4):241–50.
18. Wakili R, Voigt N, Kääb S, et al. Recent advances in the molecular pathophysiology of atrial fibrillation. J Clin Invest. 2011;121(8): 2955–68.
19. Yang Y, Xia M, Jin Q, et al. Identification of a KCNE2 gain-of-function mutation in patients with familial atrial fibrillation. Am J Hum Genet. 2004;75:899–905.
20. Fatini C, Sticchi E, Genuardi M, et al. Analysis of minK and eNOS genes as candidate loci for predisposition to non-valvular atrial fibrillation. Eur Heart J. 2006;27(14):1712–8.
21. Ma KJ, Li N, Teng SY, et al. Modulation of KCNQ1 current by atrial fibrillation-associated KCNE4 (145E/D) gene polymorphism. Chin Med J (Engl). 2007;120(2):150–4.
22. Ravn LS, Hofman-Bang J, Dixen U, et al. Relation of 97T polymorphism in KCNE5 to risk of atrial fibrillation. Am J Cardiol. 2005;96(3):405–7.
23. Olson TM, Michels VV, Ballew JD, et al. Sodium channel mutations and susceptibility to heart failure and atrial fibrillation. JAMA. 2005;293(4):447–54.
24. Watanabe H, Darbar D, Kaiser DW, et al. Mutations in sodium channel beta1- and beta2-subunits associated with atrial fibrillation. Circ Arrhythm Electrophysiol. 2009;2(3):268–75.
25. Bedi M, McNamara D, London B, et al. Genetic susceptibility to atrial fibrillation in patients with congestive heart failure. Heart Rhythm. 2006;3(7):808–12.
26. Hagendorff A, Schumacher B, Kirchhoff S, et al. Conduction disturbances and increased atrial vulnerability in Connexin40-deficient

mice analyzed by transesophageal stimulation. Circulation. 1999;99(11):1508–15.

27. Gollob MH, Jones DL, Krahn AD, et al. Somatic mutations in the connexin 40 gene (GJA5) in atrial fibrillation. N Engl J Med. 2006;54(25):2677–88.

28. Li DQ, Feng YB, Zhang HQ. The relationship between gap junctional remodeling and atrial fibrillation in patients with rheumatic heart disease. Zhonghua Yi Xue Za Zhi (abstract). 2004;84(5): 384–6.

29. Tziakas DN, Chalikias GK, Stakos DA, et al. Effect of angiotensin-converting enzyme insertion/deletion genotype on collagen type I synthesis and degradation in patients with atrial fibrillation and arterial hypertension. Expert Opin Pharmacother. 2007;8(14): 2225–34.

30. Cao FF, Chen XD, Wang QS, et al. Associations of the genetic polymorphisms in CYP11B2 gene with nonfamilial structural atrial fibrillation. Zhonghua Liu Xing Bing Xue Za Zhi (abstract). 2009;30(10):1069–72.

31. Wang QS, Li YG, Chen XD, et al. Angiotensinogen polymorphisms and acquired atrial fibrillation in Chinese. J Electrocardiol. 2010;43(4):373–7.

32. Gai X, Lan X, Luo Z, et al. Association of MMP-9 gene polymorphisms with atrial fibrillation in hypertensive heart disease patients. Clin Chim Acta. 2009;408(1–2):105–9.

33. Gai X, Zhang Z, Liang Y, et al. MMP-2 and TIMP-2 gene polymorphisms and susceptibility to atrial fibrillation in Chinese Han patients with hypertensive heart disease. Clin Chim Acta. 2010;411(9–10):719–24.

34. Gudbjartsson DF, Arnar DO, Helgadottir A, et al. Variants conferring risk of atrial fibrillation on chromosome 4q25. Nature. 2007;448:353–7.

35. Gudbjartsson DF, Holm H, Gretarsdottir S, et al. A sequence variant in ZFHX3 on 16q22 associates with atrial fibrillation and ischemic stroke. Nat Genet. 2009;41:876–8.

36. Chinchilla A, Daimi H, Lozano-Velasco E, et al. Pitx2 insufficiency leads to atrial electrical and structural remodelling linked to arrhythmogenesis. Circ Cardiovasc Genet. 2011;4(3):269–79.

37. Tessari A, Pietrobon M, Notte A, et al. Myocardial Pitx2 differentially regulates the left atrial identity and ventricular asymmetric remodeling programs. Circ Res. 2008;102(7):813–22.

38. Wang J, Klysik E, Sood S, et al. Pitx2 prevents susceptibility to atrial arrhythmias by inhibiting leftsided pacemaker specification. Proc Natl Acad Sci U S A. 2010;107(21):9753–8.

39. Kirchhof P, Khar PC, Kaese S, et al. PITX2c is expressed in the adult left atrium, and reducing Pitx2c expression promotes atrial fibrillation inducibility and complex changes in gene expression. Circ Cardiovasc Genet. 2011;4(2):123–33.

40. Lozano-Velasco E, Chinchilla A, Martinez-Fernandez S, et al. Pitx2c modulates cardiac specific transcription factor networks in differentiating cardiomyocytes from murine embryonic stem cells. Cells Tissues Organs. 2011;194(5):349–62.

41. Hjalt TA, Amendt BA, Murray JC. PITX2 regulates procollagen lysyl hydroxylase (PLOD) gene expression: implications for the pathology of Rieger syndrome. J Cell Biol. 2001;152(3):545–52.

42. Barth AS, Merk S, Arnoldi E, et al. Reprogramming of the human atrial transcriptome in permanent atrial fibrillation: expression of a ventricular-like genomic signature. Circ Res. 2005;96:1022–9.

43. Smith ML, Joglar JA, Wasmund SL, et al. Reflex control of sympathetic activity during simulated ventricular tachycardia in humans. Circulation. 1999;100:628–34.

44. Bouzegrhane F, Thibault G. Is angiotensin II a proliferative factor of cardiac fibroblasts? Cardiovasc Res. 2002;53(2):304–12.

45. Dhein S, Polontchouk L, Salameh A, et al. Pharmacological modulation and differential regulation of the cardiac gap junction proteins connexin 43 and connexin 40. Biol Cell. 2002;94(7–8):409–22.

46. Shinagawa K, Shi YF, Tardif JC, et al. Dynamic nature of atrial fibrillation substrate during development and reversal of heart failure in dogs. Circulation. 2002;105:2672–8.

47. Anyukhovsky EP, Sosunov EA, Plotnikov A, et al. Cellular electrophysiologic properties of old canine atria provide a substrate for arrhythmogenesis. Cardiovasc Res. 2005;54:462–9.

48. Kistler PM, Sanders P, Dodic M, et al. Atrial electrical and structural abnormalities in an ovine model of chronic blood pressure elevation after prenatal corticosteroid exposure: implications for development of atrial fibrillation. Eur Heart J. 2006;27:3045–56.

49. Wang TJ, Parise H, Levy D, et al. Obesity and the risk of new-onset atrial fibrillation. JAMA. 2004;292:2471–7.

50. Xiao HD, Fuchs S, Campbell DJ, et al. Mice with cardiac-restricted angiotensin-converting enzyme (ACE) have atrial enlargement, cardiac arrhythmia, and sudden death. Am J Pathol. 2004;165:1019–32.

51. Li D, Shinagawa K, Pang L, et al. Effects of angiotensin-converting enzyme inhibition on the development of the atrial fibrillation substrate in dogs with ventricular tachypacing-induced congestive heart failure. Circulation. 2001;104:2608–14.

52. Okazaki H, Minamino T, Tsukamoto O, et al. Angiotensin II type 1 receptor blocker prevents atrial structural remodeling in rats with hypertension induced by chronic nitric oxide inhibition. Hypertens Res. 2006;29:277–84.

53. Anand K, Mooss AN, Hee TT, et al. Meta-analysis: inhibition of rennin-angiotensin system prevents new-onset atrial fibrillation. Am Heart J. 2006;152:217–22.

54. Fang WT, Li HJ, Zhang H, et al. The role of statin therapy in the prevention of atrial fibrillation: a meta-analysis of randomized controlled trials. Br J Clin Pharmacol. 2012;74(5):744–56.

55. Khawaja O, Gaziano JM, Djoussé L. A meta-analysis of omega-3 Fatty acids and incidence of atrial fibrillation. J Am Coll Nutr. 2012;31(1):4–13.
56. Kaneko N. New 1,4-benzothiazepine derivative, K201, demonstrates cardioprotective effects against sudden cardiac cell death and intra-cellular calcium blocking action. Drug Dev Res. 1994;33(4):429–38.
57. Kohno M, Yano M, Kobayashi S, et al. A new cardioprotective agent, JTV519, improves defective channel gating of ryanodine receptor in heart failure. Am J Physiol Heart Circ Physiol. 2003;284(3): H1035–42.
58. Hilliard FA, Steele DS, Laver D, et al. Flecainide inhibits arrhythmo-genic Ca2+ waves by open state block of ryanodine receptor Ca2+ release channels and reduction of Ca2+ spark mass. J Mol Cell Cardiol. 2010;48:293–301.
59. Neef S, Dybkova N, Sossalla S, et al. CaMKII-dependent diastolic SR Ca2+ leak and elevated diastolic Ca2+ levels in right atrial myo-cardium of patients with atrial fibrillation. Circ Res. 2010;106: 1134–44.
60. Dobrev D, Nattel S. Calcium handling abnormalities in atrial fibril-lation as a target for innovative therapeutics. J Cardiovasc Pharmacol. 2008;52:293–9.
61. Dobrev D. Cardiomyocyte Ca2+ overload in atrial tachycardia: is blockade of L-type Ca2+ channels a promising approach to prevent electrical remodeling and arrhythmogenesis? Naunyn Schmiedebergs Arch Pharmacol. 2007;376:227–30.
62. Blomström-Lundqvist C, Blomström P. Safety and efficacy of phar-macological cardioversion of atrial fibrillation using intravenous vernakalant, a new antiarrhythmic drug with atrial selectivity. Expert Opin Drug Saf. 2012;11(4):671–9.
63. Shiroshita-Takeshita A, Sakabe M, Haugan K, et al. Model-dependent effects of the gap junction conduction-enhancing antiar-rhythmic peptide rotigaptide (ZP123) on experimental atrial fibrillation in dogs. Circulation. 2007;115:310–8.

Chapter 3
Novel Oral Anticoagulants for Stroke Prevention in Patients with Non-valvular Atrial Fibrillation

Yoseph Rozenman and Yuri Gluzman

Introduction

Atrial fibrillation (AF) is the cause of ischemic stroke in approximately 20 % of patients with stroke [1]. As compared with other etiologies stroke in patients with AF is associated with higher mortality, severe disability and high recurrence rate. Antithrombotic therapy is effective to prevent stroke in AF patients. Vitamin K Antagonists (VKA) are much more effective than aspirin and, in the absence of contraindication, are highly recommended for the majority of these patients [1, 2]. However, warfarin (a VKA) have numerous limitations (narrow therapeutic range, multiple interactions with diet and other medications, complex individualized dosing, delayed onset of action, etc.), which complicate its use [1, 2]. Target International Normalized Ratio (INR) is determined by the balance between the risk of thrombotic events and that of the catastrophic intracranial bleed. Stable therapeutic anticoagulation requires multiple blood tests and is very often hard to achieve, leading to

Y. Rozenman, MSc, MD, FACC (✉) • Y. Gluzman
Heart Institute, Edith Wolfson Medical Center, 58100 Holon, Israel

Sackler Faculty of Medicine, Tel-Aviv University, Tel Aviv, Israel
e-mail: rozenman@wolfson.health.gov.il

G.-A. Dan et al. (eds.), *Atrial Fibrillation Therapy*, Current
Cardiovascular Therapy, DOI 10.1007/978-1-4471-5475-4_3,
© Springer-Verlag London 2014

suboptimal balance between thrombosis and bleeding. Novel Oral Anticoagulants (NOACs) were developed to overcome these limitations [3, 4]. The NOACs are divided into two classes: the oral direct thrombin inhibitors (e.g. dabigatran) and oral direct factor Xa inhibitors (e.g. rivaroxaban, apixaban and edoxaban). These agents inhibit a single step in coagulation, at major variance from warfarin, which block the formation of multiple vitamin K-dependent coagulation factors (II, VII, IX, and X).

Phase III Trials of NOACs in Atrial Fibrillation

(a) **RE-LY:** The RE-LY (Randomised Evaluation of Long term anticoagulant therapY) trial was a prospective, randomized, open-label clinical phase III trial comparing two blinded doses of dabigatran (110 mg BID or 150 mg BID) with open-label, adjusted-dose warfarin aiming for a target INR of 2.0–3.0 [5]. A total of 18,113 patients with non-valvular AF and at least one risk factor for stroke (congestive heart failure, hypertension, age ≥75 years, diabetes and previous stroke – CHADS) were included. The primary outcome was stroke or systemic embolism and median treatment duration was 2 years. The rates of discontinuation at 2 years were higher with dabigatran 150 mg (20.7 %) and dabigatran 110 mg (21.2 %) than with warfarin (16.6 %). The mean and median times in therapeutic range (TTR) for warfarin treated patients were 64 % and 67 %, respectively.

There was a reduction of the primary outcome of stroke or systemic embolism from 1.69 %/year with warfarin to 1.53 %/year with dabigatran 110 mg (RR: 0.91, 0.74–1.11; p for noninferiority <0.001) and 1.11 %/year with dabigatran 150 mg (RR: 0.66, 0.53–0.82; p for superiority <0.001). The rates of hemorrhagic stroke and intracranial bleeding were significantly lower with dabigatran (0.1 %/year for both doses) compared with warfarin

(0.4 %/year; p<0.001). Gastrointestinal bleeding was increased from 1.0 %/year with warfarin to 1.5 %/year with dabigatran 150 (p<0.001). There was a non-significant increase in rate of myocardial infarction with both dabigatran doses [6]. Annual total mortality was 4.13 % for warfarin compared with 3.75 % for dabigatran 110 mg (p=0.13) and 3.64 % for dabigatran 150 mg (p=0.051). Previous VKA exposure did not influence the benefits of dabigatran at either dose, compared with warfarin [7].

The conclusions were that in patients with non-valvular AF at risk for stroke, dabigatran 150 mg BID was superior to warfarin, with no significant difference in the primary safety endpoint of major bleeding, whereas dabigatran 110 mg BID was non-inferior to warfarin, with 20 % fewer major bleeds. The rate of hemorrhagic stroke was reduced with both doses of dabigatran. Based on these results, dabigatran has been approved by the Food and Drug Administration (FDA), the European Medicines Agency (EMA) and health authorities in many countries worldwide as an alternative to warfarin for prevention of stroke and systemic embolism in patients with non-valvular AF. The FDA has approved the 150 mg dose, and the 75 mg BID dose in patients with severe renal impairment (creatinine clearance (CrCl) of 15–30 mL/min), while the EMA has approved both the 110 and 150 mg doses. Dabigatran 75 mg BID was not evaluated in the RE-LY (patients with a CrCl of <30 mL/min were excluded) and the recommendation is based on pharmacokinetic and pharmacodynamic modeling. There are no dosing recommendations for patients with CrCl<15 mL/min or patients on chronic hemodialysis.

(b) **ROCKET-AF:** The ROCKET-AF (Rivaroxaban Once Daily Oral Direct Factor Xa Inhibition Compared With Vitamin K Antagonism for Prevention of Stroke and Embolism Trial in AF) [8] is a randomized, double-blind, double-dummy study of 14,264 patients with non-valvular AF at high risk of stroke (CHADS$_2$ score of 2 or higher – mean 3.5). Patients were randomly assigned to receive either rivaroxaban 20 mg daily (15 mg for patients with renal impairment and CrCl of 30–49 mL/min) or warfarin aiming for a target INR of 2–3. The primary outcome was noninferiority of rivaroxaban versus warfarin for the occurrence of stroke or systemic embolism. Median follow-up duration was 2 years. The mean TTR for the warfarin-treated patients was 55 % (median 58 %); lower than in other NOAC randomized trials (Table 3.1). Discontinuation rate was higher with rivaroxaban (23.9 %) than with warfarin (22.4 %).

Rivaroxaban was noninferior to warfarin for the primary endpoint of stroke and systemic embolism with yearly event rate of 2.1 %, compared to 2.4 % in the warfarin group (HR with rivaroxaban: 0.88; 95 % CI: 0.75–1.03; $p < 0.001$ for noninferiority). However, using intention-to-treat analysis, rivaroxaban was not statistically superior to warfarin ($p = 0.12$). There was a non significant reduction in mortality (1.9 %/year for rivaroxaban and 2.2 %/year for warfarin, (HR: 0.85; 0.70–1.02; $P = 0.07$) or ischemic stroke, but a significant reduction in intracranial bleeding (0.5 %/year with rivaroxaban vs. 0.7 %/year with warfarin; $p = 0.02$). The yearly rate of major and non-major bleeding was not significantly different between groups (3.6 % for rivaroxaban and 3.4 % for warfarin, $p = 0.58$). There was, however, a significant reduction in fatal bleeding with rivaroxaban (0.2 %/year vs.0.5 %/year; $p = 0.003$), despite an increase in gastrointestinal bleeds and bleeds requiring transfusion (1.65 with rivaroxaban vs. 1.32 with warfarin; $p = 0.044$).

ROCKET-AF conclusion was that rivaroxaban was noninferior to warfarin for the primary endpoint of stroke and systemic embolism in high risk patients with nonvalvular AF, without increasing in the risk of major bleeding. Rivaroxaban has been approved for stroke prevention in non-valvular AF by the FDA, the EMA and in many countries worldwide.

(c) **AVERROES:** Efficacy and safety of apixaban for stroke prevention in patients with nonvalvular AF as compared to aspirin and warfarin were examined in two randomized,

TABLE 3.1 Phase III trials of NOACs: pharmacologic properties, study design and patient characteristics

	Dabigatran	Rivaroxaban	Apixaban
Target – factor	IIa	Xa	Xa
Peak level (hours)	3	3	3
Half-life (hours)	12–17	5–13	9–14
Renal elimination	80 %	33 %	25 %
Phase III study	**RE-LY**	**ROCKET-AF**	**ARISTOTLE**
Primary endpoint	Stroke (ischemic or hemorrhagic) or systemic embolism		
Safety endpoint	Major bleeding (ISTH)[a]		
Dose (mg) frequency	150,110 BID	20 (15[b]) QD	5 (2.5[b]) BID
N	18,111	14,264	18,201
Design	PROBE	Double blind	Double blind
CHADS$_2$ ≥3 (%)	32	87	30
Mean TTR (%)	64	55	62

PROBE prospective, randomized, open-label, blinded end point evaluation

[a]ROCKET – major and clinically relevant non-major bleeding

[b]Dose adjusted in patients with ↓drug clearance and other study defined characteristics

double-blind, double-dummy, phase III trials as follows: The AVERROES (Apixaban VERsus acetylsalicylic acid to pRevent strOkE in atrial fibrillation patientS who have failed or are unsuitable for warfarin) trial [9] randomized 5,599 patients with AF and at least one risk factor for stroke, who were unsuitable candidates for (or were unwilling to take) warfarin, to treatment with either apixaban 5 mg BID (2.5 mg BID in patients ≥80 years, weight ≤60 kg or with a serum creatinine ≥1.5 mg/dL) or aspirin at dose 81–324 mg/day. The study population and primary endpoint were similar to the RE-LY trial. Interestingly the rates of drug discontinuation were higher for aspirin (20.5 %/year) than for apixaban (17.9 %/year). The trial was stopped early after 1.1-year median follow-up because of a clear benefit of apixaban. There was a reduction in the rate of stroke and systemic embolism from 3.7 %/year with aspirin to 1.6 %/year with apixaban (HR: 0.45; 95 % CI: 0.32–0.62; p<0.001). Annual mortality was reduced from 4.4 % with aspirin to 3.5 % with apixaban (p=0.07) and there was no significant difference in rates of major bleeding (1.2 %/year with aspirin vs. 1.4 %/year with apixaban, p=0.57) or intracranial bleeding (0.4 %/year in both groups). The conclusions was that in patients with non-valvular AF at risk for stroke, apixaban treatment associated with a 55 % reduction in ischemic stroke or systemic embolism compared to aspirin without significantly increasing the risk of major or intracranial bleeding.

(d) **ARISTOTLE**: (Apixaban for Reduction of Stroke and Other Thromboembolic Events in AF) trial [10] compared apixaban 5 mg BID (2.5 mg BID in patients ≥80 years, weight ≤60 kg or with a serum creatinine ≥1.5 mg/dL) to warfarin aiming for a target INR of 2–3 in 18,201 patients with non-valvular AF documented in the 12 months before randomization and at least one additional risk factor for stroke (CHADS$_2$ score 1 or higher, mean 2.1). The study population was similar to the study populations in the AVERROES and RE-LY trials. The primary efficacy outcome was stroke or systemic embolism and the primary safety outcome was major bleeding. Median treatment duration was 1.8 years with a minimum of 1-year follow-up. The mean TTR for the warfarin treated patients was 62.2 % (median 66 %). Discontinuation due to adverse reactions was higher with warfarin (27.5 %) than with apixaban (25.3 %).

There was a reduction of the primary outcome of stroke or systemic embolism from 1.60 %/year with warfarin to 1.27 %/year with apixaban (HR: 0.79; 95 % CI: 0.66–0.95; p=0.01 for superiority) without significant difference in incidence of ischemic stroke. The rate of major bleeding was 3.09 %/year for warfarin compared with 2.13 %/year for apixaban (p < 0.001). Rates of hemorrhagic stroke and intracranial bleeding were significantly lower with apixaban (0.33 %/year) than with warfarin (0.80 %/year, p < 0.001). Gastrointestinal bleeding was not statistically different between treatments (0.86 %/year for warfarin, 0.76 %/for apixaban) – a finding that is unique for apixaban (see RE-LY and ROCKET-AF trials), Total mortality was significantly reduced by apixaban: 3.94 %/year for warfarin compared with 3.52 %/year for apixaban (p = 0.047).

It was thus concluded that apixaban treatment in patients with non-valvular AF and increased risk of stroke is associated with a 21 % reduction in ischemic stroke or systemic embolism, 31 % reduction in major bleeding and 11 % reduction in all-cause mortality compared to warfarin. Apixaban has been approved recently for stroke prevention in nonvalvular AF by the FDA, the EMA and in many countries worldwide.

Between Trial Comparison

(a) **Pharmacologic properties and design differences:** Table 3.1 describes the pharmacologic properties of the three currently available NOACs [3]. Dabigatran inhibits factor IIa while rivaroxaban and apixaban inhibit factor Xa. Time to peak plasma concentration and half life are very similar for the three agents. Dabigatran, as compared to rivaroxaban and apixaban, is cleared from the circulation mostly by the kidney. Primary and safety trial endpoints were similar however, despite the similarities in the pharmacologic properties there is marked variation in study designs. Since this variation is not explained by pharmacokinetic differenced it reflects an attempt by the investigators to choose dosing scheme that will optimize the balance between efficacy and safety; a decision that was based on theoretical assumptions and results of preliminary trials.

The RE-LY investigators [4, 5] compared two separate drug doses without dose adjustment to renal function (patients with CrCl < 30 mL/min were excluded) even though dabigatran plasma level is expected to be influenced by renal function more than the anti Xa agents. It was the RE-LY investigators hope that the identification of two doses with similar efficacy as adjusted dose warfarin might provide an opportunity to tailor the dose to individual patients to maximize the benefit against risk. In ROCKET-AF [8, 11], rivaroxaban dose was reduced by 25 % in patients with impaired renal function (CrCl of 30–49 mL/min) while in ARISTOTLE [10, 12], apixaban dose was reduced by 50 % in those with impaired function or those who were judged to be at high bleeding risk (two of the following criteria: age $\geq$80 years, a body weight <60 kg, and a serum creatinine level $\geq$1.5 mg/dL).

Despite similar half life ROCKET-AF investigators elected to choose once daily drug schedule that initially seems inappropriate for a drug with half life 5–13 h. This decision was based on dose finding preliminary trials [13] in which the same total daily doses given once daily achieved, on the average, higher maximum plasma concentration values (~20 %) and lower trough concentrations (~60 %) than when given twice daily, however, the 5th–95th percentile ranges for these parameters overlapped. Moreover, Weitz et al. [14] conducted a dose finding trial with edoxaban in patients with AF and concluded that for the same total daily dose of 60 mg, both bleeding frequency and trough edoxaban concentrations were higher in the 30-mg BID group than in the 60-mg QD group. These results emphasize the complexity of our ability to predict efficacy and bleeding based on pharmacokinetic information. The balance between efficacy and safety and the optimal diurnal variation of plasma levels (including peak and trough values) might vary among indications and organs. Bleeding may theoretically be prevented by lower trough value [14] even if peak levels are high. Low trough value might however be associated with the creation of a small clot that might cause the clinical event or might dissolve at the time of a high peak level (QD dosing) before becoming clinically significant. Thus the optimal dose and dosing schedule may vary with the clinical indication.

Double blind randomized trial is the accepted standard in phase III drug evaluation trials. Whether PROBE (prospective, randomized, open-label, blinded end point evaluation) design provides a more realistic comparison to warfarin is a subject of debate.

(b) **Results:** Table 3.2 describes the outcome of the three NOACs as compared to warfarin. Before any conclusion can be made regarding the assessment of the comparative safety and effectiveness of the three NOACs it is worthwhile to look at the outcomes in the warfarin groups of these trials. The rate of stroke or systemic embolism (primary endpoint) in ROCKET-AF was approximately 50 % higher than the rates observed in ARISTOTLE or RE-LY. This difference may be explained by differences in patient's characteristics or in the quality of care among trials. In fact ROCKET-AF design guaranteed enrollment of patients at much higher stroke risk. TTR is considered as an accepted surrogate for quality of care and mean TTR value in ROCKET-AF was 55 % (lower than 64 % and 62 % in ARISTOTLE and RE-LY respectively). However apart from quality of care TTR values are also influenced by patient's characteristics (sicker patients with higher $CHADS_2$ score in ROCKET-AF), the exact application of the Rosendaal method [15] and study design (PROBE vs. double blind).

The main conclusion from a formal indirect comparison among trials using the Bucher method [16] was that there are no profound significant differences in efficacy between apixaban and dabigatran (both doses) or rivaroxaban. Dabigatran 150 mg BID was superior to rivaroxaban for efficacy (with less stroke and systemic embolism). Major

Table 3.2 Trial outcome of phase III trials of NOACs (From Camm et al. [3] with permission)

Outcomes (% per year)	RE-LY			ROCKET-AF		ARISTOTLE	
	Warfarin	Dabigatran 150	Dabigatran 110	Warfarin	Rivaroxaban	Warfarin	Apixaban
	(n=6,022)	(n=6,076)	(n=6,015)	(n=1)	(n=7,131)	(n=9,0811)	(n=9,120)
		(RR, 95 % CI; P value)	(RR, 95 % CI; P value)		(HR, 95 % CI; P value)		(HR, 95 % CI; P value)
Stroke/systemic embolism	1.69	1.11 (0.66. 0.53–0.82; P for superiority <0.001)	1.53(0.91. 0.74–1.11; P for non-inferiority <0.001)	2.4	2.1 (0.88, 0.75–1.03; P for non-Inferiority <0.0001, P for superiority=0.12) (ITT)	1.6	1.27 (0.79, 0.66–0.95; P<0.001 for non-Inferiority, P=0.01 for superiority)
Ischaemic stroke	1.2	0.92 (0.76, 0.60–0.98; P=0.03)	1.34 (1.11, 0.89–1.40; P=0.35)	1.42	1.34 (0.94;0.75–1.17; P=0.581)	1.05	0.97 (0.92, 0.74–1.13; P=0.42)
Haemorrhagic stroke	0.38	0.10 (0.26, 0.14–0.49; P<0.001)	0.12 (0.31, 0.17–0.56; P<0.001)	0.44	0.26 (0.59; 0.37–0.93; P=0.024)	0.47	0.24 (0.51, 0.35–0.75; P<0.001)
Major bleeding	3.36	3.11 (0.93, 0.81–1.07; P=0.31)	2.71 (0.80, 0.69–0.93; P=0.003)	3.4	3.6 (P=0.58)	3.09	2.13 (0.69,0.60–0.80; P<0.001)

Intracranial bleeding	0.74	0.30 (0.40, 0.27–0.60; $P<0.001$)	0.23 (0.31, 0.20–0.47; $P<0.001$)	0.7	0.5 (0.67; 0.47–0.93; $P=0.02$)	0.80	0.33(0.42, 0.30–0.58; $P<0.001$)
Extracranial bleeding	2.67	2.84 (1.07, 0.92–1.25; $P=0.38$)	2.51 (0.94, 0.80–1.10; $P=0.45$)	–	–	–	–
Gastrointestinal bleeding	1.02	1.51 (1.50, 1.19–1.89; $P<0.001$)	1.12 (1.10, 0.86–1.41; $P=0.43$)	2.2	3.2 ($P<0.001$)	0.86	0.76 (0.89, 0.70–1.15; $P=0.37$)
Myocardial infarction	0.64	0.81 (1.27, 0.94–1.71; $P=0.12$)	0.82 (1.29, 096–1.75; $P=0.09$)	1.1	0.9 (0.81; 0.63–1.06; $P=0.12$)	0.61	0.53 (0.88, 0.66–1.17; $P=0.37$)
Death from any cause	4.13	3.64 (0.88, 0.77–1.00; $P=0.051$)	3.75 (0.91, 0.80–1.03; $P=0.13$)	2.2	1.9 (0.85; 0.70–1.02; $P=0.07$)	3.94	3.52 (0.89, 0.80–0.99; $P=0.047$)
% Discontinuation at the end of follow-up	10.2	15.5	14.5	22.2	23.7	27.5	25.3
% Discontinuation/year	5.1	7.8	7.3	11.7	12.5	15.3	14.1

Ref: [3]

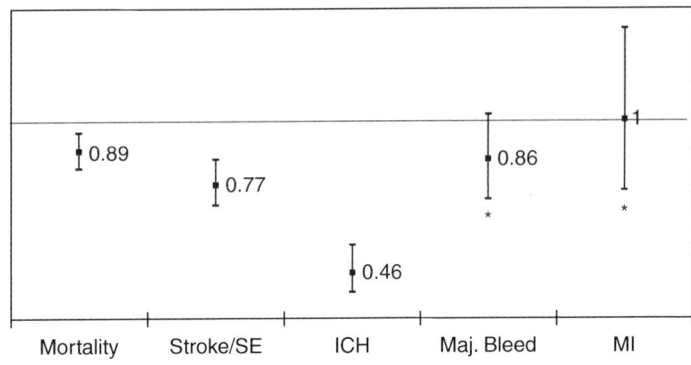

FIGURE 3.1 Relative risk of NOACs versus warfarin – Meta-analysis of randomized trials [9]. *SE* systemic embolism, *ICH* intracranial hemorrhage, *MI* Myocardial infarction, * Heterogeneity among trials

bleeding was lower with dabigatran 110 mg BID or apixaban. Rates of myocardial infarction were higher with dabigatran especially when compared with rivaroxaban. However, as the authors state, differences in inclusion and exclusion criteria, patient population, data collection methods, and outcome definitions or adjudication could result in residual confounding factors that can potentially explain these observed differences.

Since there are more similarities than differences a meta-analysis is appropriate to provide a reliable estimation of the benefit of NOACs as compared to warfarin. Such meta-analysis [17] retrieved data from 12 studies enrolling 54,875 patients (Fig. 3.1). NOACs significantly reduced total mortality (RR 0.89; 95 % CI, 0.83–0.96), cardiovascular mortality (RR 0.89; 95 % CI, 0.82–0.98) and stroke or systemic embolism (RR 0.77; 95 % CI, 0.70–0.86). There was a trend towards reduced major bleeding (RR 0.86; 95 % CI, 0.72–1.02), with a significant reduction of intracranial hemorrhage (RR 0.46; 95 % CI, 0.39–0.56). No difference in myocardial infarction was observed (RR 1.00; 95 % CI, 0.75–1.33). There was some heterogeneity among trials in major bleeding and rates of myocardial infarction that might reflect variation in patient characteristics, study designs or drug (dose) effects.

NOACs in Coronary Artery Disease

A generally accepted "rule" in antithrombotic therapy for patients with heart disease is that anticoagulation is more effective than antiplatelet therapy for stroke prevention in patients with AF while the opposite is true for treating patients with coronary artery disease. In fact this division between the clotting cascade and the platelets is an oversimplification since these processes are closely correlated and the most potent stimulant of platelets is thrombin [18]. Blocking thrombin, regardless of the mechanism, indirectly block platelets so that the intensity of antiplatelet therapy can be reduced in those who are adequately anticoagulated. Warfarin, as compared to placebo reduces the risks of death, reinfarction or stroke [19] and is at least as effective as aspirin for post myocardial infarction secondary prevention [20]. Based on these data warfarin (without an antiplatelet drug) is currently recommend [21, 22] for treatment of patients with AF and stable coronary artery disease. Whether this recommendation can be extended to NOACs is not clear. It is also not entirely clear whether anti Xa provide different protection from cardiac events as compared to anti IIa.

Between 10 % and 15 % of patients with acute coronary syndrome suffer also from AF (or develop it during hospitalization). Patients with acute coronary syndrome are usually treated with dual anti platelet therapy and the majority of them undergo stent implantation. Since aspirin and clopidogrel are not effective enough to prevent stroke in patients with AF [23] warfarin is added so that they are treated with "triple antithrombotic regimen" exposing them to high bleeding risk [24]. Recently a small trial (573 patients) randomized patients on warfarin who underwent stent implantation to addition of clopidogrel or standard addition of aspirin and clopidogrel [25]. Bleeding, as expected, was significantly reduced while the combined secondary endpoint of thrombotic events (including stent thrombosis) was not compromised and there was a significant reduction in mortality. As much as this data is reassuring it is not sufficient (lack of power) to recommend avoiding aspirin in these patients. Current recommendations advice using "triple therapy" in these patients adjusting warfarin to low therapeutic range and determining the duration of combined treatment based on clinical presentation (stable patients or acute coronary syndrome), type of stent implanted (bare metal drug eluting of first or second generation) and the assessment of the individual bleeding risk [19, 20].

Modern therapy of patients with AF prefers the use of NOACs as an alternative to warfarin. In patients with acute coronary syndrome newer antiplatelets (prasugrel or ticagrelor) are preferred over clopidogrel. Despite the large number of patients with AF and acute coronary syndrome the optimal antithrombotic therapy in these patients is unknown since they were usually excluded from both AF and acute coronary syndrome trials. There is absolutely no data on the combined use of NOACs with either prasugrel or ticagrelor. Based on animal data that showed reduction of thrombus weight by rivaroxaban in a stent thrombosis model [26] a large phase III trial showed that the addition of low dose rivaroxaban to the standard combination of aspirin and clopidogrel is associated with significant reduction in cardiovascular events stent thrombosis and mortality [27]. There is however no data on the effect of standard rivaroxaban dose and in fact patients with AF were excluded from this trial. Post-hoc analysis of the RE-LY trial suggests, based on a limited number of patients, that dabigatran combined with dual antiplatelet therapy maintains its advantages over warfarin [28] – specifically dabigatran 110 BID is associated with lower bleeding rate than warfarin in patients on a combination of two antiplatelet agents. No such data are available for rivaroxaban and apixaban since patients on dual antiplatelet therapy were excluded from ROCKET-AF and ARISTOTLE. Since there is no or insufficient data on the combination of the new antiplatelet agents with warfarin, or on NOACs in combination with aspirin and clopidogrel, current recommendation is to use "old" triple therapy with aspirin clopidogrel and warfarin leaving this large group of patients with therapy that might be inferior to those without this combination. Since many physicians are uncomfortable with this recommendation, local practice may vary among centers despite the lack of clinical evidence. There is thus an urgent need for trials to clarify the role of NOACs and new antiplatelet agents in this important group of patients.

Thrombosis and Bleeding: Relation to Mechanism of Action

Pharmacokinetic information and in-vitro tests are helpful to analyze the effect of NOACs but due to the complexity of the pathophysiology of bleeding and thrombosis are the true safety and efficacy can be determined only from large clinical trials. The balance between efficacy and safety might vary among organs (atria, deep veins, brain, gastrointestinal tract etc.) and the optimal diurnal variation of plasma levels (including peak and trough concentrations) may vary among indications and organs. Theoretically, assuming that the majority of bleeding events are triggered by vessel trauma (usually spontaneous), stable "mild" anticoagulation might be associated with slow continuous bleed that stops at a time of "under-anticoagulation" (association between trough level and safety) [14]. On the efficacy side, low trough value might theoretically be associated with the creation of a small clot that will be later dissolved at the time of a high peak level (QD dosing). This small clot might be tolerated in the deep veins or in the atria but not in a coronary artery.

Dabigatran 150 mg BID is associated with higher rate of gastrointestinal bleed as compared to warfarin ($RR=1.5$, $p<0.001$) but less intracranial bleed ($RR=0.30$, $p<0.01$). Dabigatran 150 BID is more potent than standard dose warfarin in preventing clot formation in the atria and the associated ischemic stroke ($RR=0.92$, $p=0.03$) but is probably less effective than warfarin in preventing thrombotic complications in patients with artificial valve despite the use of higher dose (up to 300 mg BID) [29, 30]. The exact explanation of these phenomena is unclear. It is thus very unlikely than an equivalent anticoagulant dose can be defined for different agents (especially when they differ in the mechanism of action).

Weitz [31] attempted to explain these discrepancies based on the relative effect of NOACs as compared to warfarin on the initiation and propagation phases of the thrombotic process [32]. Intracranial hemostasis is mostly extravascular and is triggered by high brain concentration of tissue factor. Hemostatic plug in the brain is dependent on the accumulation of large amount of thrombin during the propagation phase. Warfarin, as a potent inhibitor of the propagation phase, prevents this accumulation and is thus associated with a higher risk of extension of intracranial hematoma [33]. Gastrointestinal bleed – surface bleed – is influenced by systemic anticoagulation but also by the active local anticoagulant activity of the NOACs in the gut which is almost absent in the case of warfarin. Plaque rupture is usually the cause of myocardial infarction and the initiation of coronary thrombosis is triggered by the release of tissue factor. Warfarin, due to its profound effect on coagulation blocks this process and effectively protects from myocardial infarction. Anti Xa agents might be more potent than anti IIa thanks to upstream blockage of the anticoagulation cascade so that stoichiometrically less molecules of anti Xa (compared to anti IIa) are needed to block similar number of thrombin molecules.

Assessment of Level of Coagulation: In-Vitro Blood Tests

The stable and reproducible pharmacokinetics of the NOACs is an advantage over VKA's, allowing them to be administered with fixed dosing, thus routine laboratory monitoring of coagulation parameters is not recommended [34–37]. Routine coagulation tests are altered in patients receiving NOACs, but their alterations reflect poorly the circulating concentrations; particularly at high concentrations of drugs [38, 39].

TABLE 3.3 Coagulation and thrombophilia parameters under NOACs therapy

Coagulation parameters	Direct thrombin inhibitors	Factor Xa inhibitors
Prothrombin time	Unaffected/↑	↑ ↑
Partial thromboplastin time	↑ ↑	↑
Thrombin time Ecarin clotting time	↑ ↑	Unaffected
Fibrinogen	Unaffected/↓	Unaffected
D-Dimer	Unaffected	Unaffected
Antithrombin FIIa-based assay	↑	Unaffected
Antithrombin FXa-based assay	Unaffected	↑
Protein C,S activity clot based	↑	↑
Protein C,S activity chromogenic	Unaffected	Unaffected
LA screen and confirm	Falsely prolonged	Falsely prolonged

LA lupus anticoagulants

Determination of anticoagulation effect and NOACs concentrations may be required in following circumstances: (a) Major bleeding complication. (b) Suspected drug failure (i.e. thrombotic event in patient on NOAC). (c) Emergency surgery or invasive procedure. (d) Non-urgent assessment of drug levels (patients with deteriorating renal function; establishing the optimal dose in patients at extreme body weights).

Detailed knowledge about these drugs' effects on routine coagulation assays is essential for clinical practice.

1. Influence of NOACs on standard coagulation assays (Table 3.3):

   • PT/INR: Not significantly influenced by direct thrombin inhibitors (dabigatran); patients can have a normal or near normal PT/INR despite having considerable dabigatran concentrations. Direct factor Xa inhibitors (rivaroxaban, apixaban) prolong the PT/INR so that this test can be useful as an estimate for the anticoagulation effect. PT is not however sensitive enough to detect clinically relevant changes in anti Xa drug concentration [40, 41].

- aPTT: Prolongation of aPTT occurs with both direct factor Xa and thrombin inhibitors, however it is more sensitive and clinically useful to estimate the effect of dabigatran. The utility of aPTT is primarily for its negative predictive value, i.e. a normal aPTT confirms mild (at most) anticoagulant activity [38, 42–44].
- Fibrinogen: Not affected by factor Xa inhibitors but dabigatran may lead to a falsely reduced concentration in some test assays [42, 45].
- Thrombin time (TT) and the Ecarin Clotting Time (ECT): highly sensitive tests for dabigatran and are useful for monitoring its activity. Factor Xa inhibitors have no impact on the TT/ECT [46].

2. Influence of NOACs on thrombophilia parameters (Table 3.3):
   Both traditional and new anticoagulants target key enzymes of the coagulation cascade. Anticoagulant therapy may interfere also with certain thrombophilia tests. Presence of NOACs causes an overestimation of protein C or S levels in clotting assays and may result in falsely prolongation of lupus anticoagulant screen [36]. Intrinsic factor assays (VIII, IX, XI, and XII) as well as other factors might also be affected however there is no large enough published data on the magnitude of this effect.

3. Direct determination of the NOACs activity (Table 3.4):
   Levels of the NOACs are best determined using diagnostic assays, which use calibrators and controls specific for the anticoagulant to be measured. Mass spectrometry can be used to measure all three drugs over a broad concentration range [47, 48]. Dabigatran can be monitored using a Hemoclot Thrombin Inhibitor Assay or an ECT assay. Apixaban and rivaroxaban can be monitored using chromogenic anti Xa assays that use specific apixaban or rivaroxaban standards.

TABLE 3.4 Qualitative and quantitative assessment of NOACs activity

	Direct Thrombin Inhibitors	Factor Xa Inhibitors
Qualitative assessment	aPTT Thrombin time	Prothrombin time*
Quantitative assessment	Hemoclot assay Ecarin clotting time	Chromogenic anti-Xa assays

aCalibrated

Conclusion: NOACs affect a variety of routine as well as special coagulation assays. The aPTT is affected more than PT by dabigatran and can be qualitatively useful to estimate its effect. Rivaroxaban and apixaban prolong the PT to a greater extent than the aPTT so that calibrated PT is qualitatively useful for their activity. Quantitative assays (such as ECT and anti Xa assay) will be available in the near future and will enable accurate assessment of anticoagulant activity of NOACs.

Approach to Bleeding

In clinical trials of NOACs, major bleeding rates were generally low and comparable to those with warfarin [5, 8–10]. Bleeding complications and lack of specific antidotes are still major concerns. Current data regarding reversal of NOACs are derived from studies in vitro or in animals and healthy human volunteers, so that their applicability bleeding patients on NOACs is very limited. A monoclonal antibody targeted against dabigatran is currently under development [49]. Plasma-derived and recombinant factor Xa are being investigated as antidotes for factor Xa inhibitors [50, 51].

Approach to actively bleeding patients include: (1) Initial assessment with attention to hemodynamic stability, level of coagulation, renal function and time elapsed since last drug dose. (2) Identification of bleeding source. (3) Bleeding risk stratification. (4) Reversal of coagulation according to bleeding risk and level of coagulation.

Since there is no currently an available antidote for NOACs, reversal strategy is based on coagulation factor administration (passive and/or activated). To achieve reversal plasma free drug concentration should be low enough so that factors (active or passive) can be given at an amount that will exceed drug inhibitory capacity. Issues of half life (drug vs. reversing agent) should be considered. The final goal is to reach a situation in which thrombin can be generated.

Available options for passive factors are as follows: (1) Fresh frozen plasma (FFP) – there is no data regarding the use of FFP in patients with NOACs associated bleeding. In mice receiving high-dose dabigatran, FFP reduced the volume of intracerebral hemorrhage, but had no effect on mortality [52]. (2) Prothrombin complex concentrates (PCC, non-activated) – contain high doses of vitamin K-dependent coagulation factors including also proteins C and S. Two forms are available: four-factor PCC (contains factors II, VII, IX, X) and three-factor PCC (contains factors II, IX, X). In healthy volunteers, a high dose of four-factor PCC (50 U/kg) reversed PT prolongation due to rivaroxaban, but did not correct aPTT prolongation due to dabigatran [53]. It is unclear whether correction of laboratory tests would correspond to amelioration of bleeding in patients.

Options of prohemostatic agents: (1) Recombinant activated factor VII (rFVIIa) – does not correct aPTT, thrombin generation, and platelet activation in healthy volunteers receiving NOAC [54]. It is unclear however whether this therapy is of benefit when emergency anticoagulation reversal is required. (2) Activated PCC (aPCC) is a coagulation complex containing activated factors II, VII, IX and X. aPCC corrects the anticoagulant effect of high dose rivaroxaban in animal models [55]. aPCC corrected also thrombin generation parameters in plasma from healthy volunteers receiving rivaroxaban, apixaban and dabigatran [56].

Urgent hemodialysis should be considered in actively bleeding patients, or in bleeding patients with renal impairment receiving dabigatran [57]. Direct Xa inhibitors are not expected to be dialyzable because of high plasma protein binding. Oral activated charcoal may be effective for reducing dabigatran absorption following recent ingestion (within 2 h) [38]. There are no data regarding the use of oral activated charcoal with direct Xa inhibitors. There are no clinical data regarding the efficacy of desmopressin, tranexamic or aminocaproic acid. These agents may be considered as adjunctive therapies in the event of severe bleeding. Protamine sulfate and vitamin K are not expected to affect NOACs induced coagulopathy.

Management of actively bleeding patient: Bleeding patient on NOACs should undergo rapid assessment of hemodynamic status and basic coagulation tests (aPTT/TT for dabigatran, PT and anti Xa activity for direct Xa inhibitors) should be obtained. Bleeding source should be identified and the risk of the patients should be determined. A normal TT (or normal aPTT if TT is unavailable) in a patient receiving dabigatran, or a normal PT and normal anti-factor Xa activity in a patient receiving rivaroxaban or apixaban suggest very low drug levels and normal hemostatic function [38, 41, 43, 58, 59].

Figure 3.2 [60] describes treatment algorithm for management of bleeding in patients receiving NOACs. Minor bleeding (e.g. epistaxis or ecchymosis) should be managed using local hemostatic measures with delaying the next dose of NOAC or drug withdrawal for a short period after balancing individual thromboembolic risk. NOACs should be discontinued in patients with moderate bleeding (e.g. gastrointestinal bleeding) and should be followed by an attempt to achieve local control by mechanical compression, local therapy or surgical intervention. Volume replacement and blood transfusion should be considered in hypovolemic patients. Administration of blood products may be useful in selected patients (FFP for correction of dilutional coagulopathy, platelets for patient receiving antiplatelet agents). Oral charcoal and hemodialysis may be considered in selected patients on dabigatran. Patients with severe or life threatening bleeding should be managed in intensive care setting with provision of life-supporting therapies

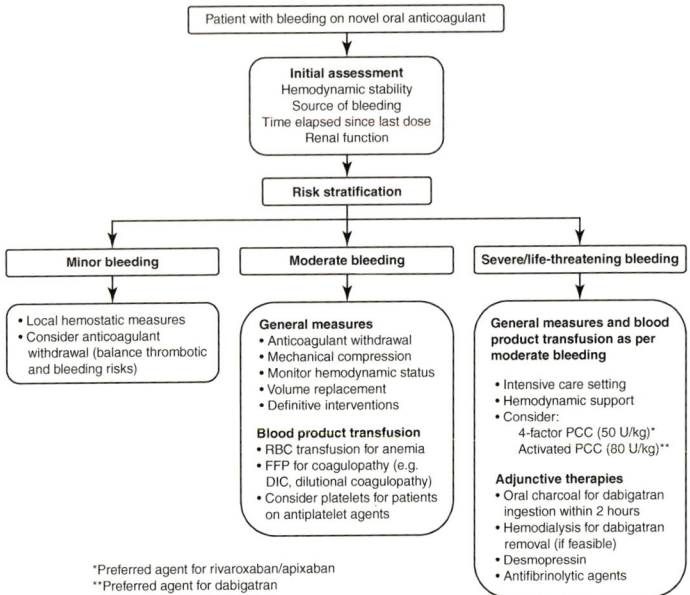

FIGURE 3.2 Suggested management of active bleeding in patient receiving NOAC (from Siegal et al. [60] with permission)

(e.g. volume replacement, blood transfusion, vasopressors, mechanical ventilation) as required. Procedural or surgical hemostasis should be achieved if possible. Administration of coagulation agents (four–factor PCC, 50 IU/kg for direct Xa inhibitors; aPCC, 80 IU/kg for dabigatran) may be reasonable [60]. Hemodialysis should be considered for dabigatran removal especially in patients with renal impairment. Adjunctive therapies such as desmopressin or antifibrinolytic agents may also be added.

Summary: Lower rate of significant bleeding is expected in patients treated with NOACs (as compared to VKAs). However, no specific antidotes are currently available to reverse their anticoagulant effect in actively bleeding patient. Drug withdrawal, aggressive supportive management and procedural/surgical hemostasis remain the mainstays of treatment. More studies are needed to clarify the role of hemostatic agents (FFP, three-factor PCC, four-factor PCC, aPCC and rFVIIa) for the reversal of the NOACs in the event of bleeding complications.

Elective/Urgent Surgery (Procedures)

(a) Surgery/Procedures

The periprocedural management of patients who are receiving long-term oral anticoagulant therapy is a very common clinical problem. It is well known that continuing oral anticoagulation is associated with an increased bleeding risk in the periprocedural period and while the absence of anticoagulant therapy for a long period preoperatively and mainly postoperatively confers a marked increased risk for stroke, systemic and venous thromboembolism, especially after major surgery [61, 62]. VKA's have a delayed onset and offset of action, requiring occasionally bridging therapy and regular monitoring of the INR that often prolongs hospitalization [63]. The emergence and routine clinical use of NOACs have the potential to simplify periprocedural anticoagulant management because of their relatively short elimination half-lives, rapid onset of action, predictable pharmacokinetic properties, and few drug interactions [64]. Given the rapid onset and offset of action of NOACs, no bridging therapy is required for the majority of interventions. Patients at extreme thrombotic risk may still require bridging with low molecular-weight or unfractionated heparin [65].

Elective procedures and surgeries: The optimal timing of NOACs discontinuation in patients who require elective procedure or surgery is determined based on three factors: (1) periprocedural bleeding risk, (2) regular elimination half-life of NOACs and (3) renal function that predicts NOACs elimination for the specific patient [64].

Procedures that appear to have a low bleeding risk (2-day risk of major bleed 0–2 %) include: Gastrointestinal endoscopy with or without biopsy, thyroid/breast/lymph node biopsies, coronary angiography, electrophysiologic testing include catheter ablation of AF, pacemaker or cardiac defribillator insertion, diagnostic bronchoscopy/hysteroscopy/cystoscopy, endosonography and arthroscopy. Surgeries with a low bleeding risk include: Nonmajor procedures (lasting less than 45 min), abdominal hernia repair, abdominal hysterectomy, cholecystectomy, cataract surgery, hemorrhoidal surgery, skin cancer excision, shoulder/foot/hand surgery and simple dental extractions [66, 67]. In cases where the ability to achieve local control of bleeding during the procedure/surgery is limited the duration of NOAC discontinuation should be increased.

Surgeries and procedures that appear to have a high bleeding risk (2-day risk of major bleed 2–4 %) include: Major cardiovascular surgery (heart valve replacement, coronary artery bypass, abdominal aortic aneurysm repair), orthopedic surgery (bilateral knee replacement, laminectomy), neurosurgery, head and neck surgery, breast cancer surgery, urologic surgery (transurethral prostate resection), kidney biopsy, polypectomy and any surgeries and procedures lasting longer than 45 min [67, 68].

Preoperative interruption of dabigatran: It is well established that dabigatran elimination half-life depends on patient's renal function: 13 h for normal renal function (CrCl>80 mL/min), 14–17 h for mild renal dysfunction (CrCl, 50–80 mL/min), 16–18 h in patients with moderate (CrCl, 30–50 mL/min) and 25 h in patients with severe (CrCl<30 mL/min) renal impairment [36, 66]. Thus before surgeries and procedures with low bleeding risk it is recommended to discontinue dabigatran for 24–48 h if renal function is normal or mildly impaired and for 48–72 h in patients with moderate renal dysfunction (CrCl 30–50 mL/min [69, 70]. There are a growing number of invasive procedures that may not require cessation of warfarin (gastrointestinal endoscopy, diagnostic bronchoscopy, coronary angiography, catheter ablation of AF, cataract extraction, pacemaker implantation). It may be reasonable also to continue dabigatran in these patients however there is currently no clinical data to support this approach. Owing to the lack of a validated antidote, a short therapeutic window of 24 h before the procedure and re-initiation of therapy 24 h after the procedure is reasonable [65]. Dabigatran should be discontinued 3 days (CrCl > 50 mL/min) or 4–5 days (CrCl < 50 mL/min) before invasive or surgical procedures with high bleeding risk [37, 38]. In high risk cases the exact timing of the procedure/surgery can be determined based on in vitro tests (aPTT or TT).

Preoperative interruption of factor Xa inhibitors: Preoperative drug interruption, like in case of dabigatran, is determined based on drug elimination half-live and the drug dependence on renal clearance. It is recommended to discontinue rivaroxaban and apixaban for 24–48 h before surgeries and procedures with low bleeding risk if renal function is normal or mildly impaired (CrCl > 50 mL/min). In patients with moderate renal dysfunction (CrCl 30-50 mL/min), it is recommended to cease rivaroxaban or apixaban for 48–72 h before the surgery. Rivaroxaban and apixaban should be discontinued 3 days (CrCl > 50 mL/min) or 4 days (CrCl < 50 mL/min) before invasive or surgical procedures with high bleeding risk [65, 71]. In high risk cases the exact timing of the procedure/surgery can be determined based on in vitro tests (PT or anti Xa level).

Postoperative resumption of new oral anticoagulants: Restarting postoperative NOACs treatment is determined by the possibility of oral administration and the risk of postoperative bleeding (related to surgery and/or the anesthetic technique). Since anticoagulation is achieved within a few hours (unlike warfarin) and since there is no available antidote therapy should be delayed until this risk has been controlled with certainty. Curative dose should not be administered before 24 h (in patients undergoing surgeries and procedures with low bleeding risk) and 48–72 h (high bleeding risk). Low-dose regimen (dabigatran 150 mg once a day, rivaroxaban 10 mg once a day or apixaban 2.5 mg once a day) for the first 2–3 days in patients undergoing high risk surgery followed by standard dose thereafter may be considered [71].

Perioperative bridging anticoagulation: As noted before, rapid onset and offset of action of NOACs should obviate the need for perioperative bridging of anticoagulation in the majority of patients. However, within the first 24–72 h after surgery, bridging therapy with a reversible anticoagulant such as unfractionated or low-molecular-weight heparin should be considered in the following conditions: (1) patients at high thrombotic risk (recurrent idiopathic venous thromboembolism, recent proximal deep venous thrombosis with or without pulmonary embolism, AF with a history of cardioembolic event), (2) patients who are unable to take oral medications, (3) patients with gastric resection or postoperative ileus in whom NOAC bioavailability may be compromised for a prolonged period [72, 73].

Emergency procedures and surgeries: Discussion with the surgeon and the anesthetist is of paramount importance in case of urgent invasive procedure or surgery in a patient receiving NOAC. Assessment of coagulation (aPTT/TT for dabigatran and PT and anti Xa for direct Xa inhibitors) and renal function should be performed. The time elapsed since last dose of drug should be obtained. NOACs should be discontinued and surgery should be postponed as long as clinically possible (at least 1–2 elimination half-lives of the drug or based on a sensitive laboratory assay) especially if surgery is of high for bleeding risk. If the patient has taken dabigatran in the preceding 2 h and there is no surgical or anesthetic contraindication, activated charcoal may be considered to reduce dabigatran absorption [38]. There are no data regarding the use of oral activated charcoal with direct Xa inhibitors. Renal perfusion and urine output should be optimized to shorten elimination half life (especially for dabigatran). Hemodialysis needs to be considered in high risk patient on dabigatran in whom postponing surgery for one or two half-lives is not clinically possible [74]. Hemodialysis is very effective, but difficult to implement in context of urgent procedure. The benefit/risk of non-specific antagonists (aPCC, rFVIIa, etc.) should be evaluated on an individual basis and, in general, these agents are not recommended as preventive measures in the absence of significant bleeding. Regional (neuraxial) anesthesia should be avoided in a patient for at least 24–48 after last NOAC dose [75].

In case of bleeding general supportive measures should be used (see section "Approach to Bleeding"). Additional hemostatic agents (three-factor PCC, four-factor PCC, aPCC or rFVIIa) may be considered during or after surgery if bleeding continues [60]. The timing of re-initiation of NOAC and the need for bridging therapy should be determined based on similar principles as in patients after elective procedures.

(b) Cardioversion and AF Ablation

Cardioversion: Although NOACs were not studied in a prospective randomized trial to assess their safety and efficacy for cardioversion data are available for dabigatran since unlike ROCKET-AF and ARISTOTLE cardioversion on dabigatran was permitted in the RELY trial. A total of 1,983 cardioversions were performed in 1,270 patients (approximately 650 procedures on warfarin and on each dabigatran dose) [76]. Stroke and systemic embolism rates at 30 days were 0.8 % (dabigatran 110 mg) 0.3 % (dabigatran 150 mg), and 0.6 % (warfarin). Major bleeding rates were 1.7 %, 0.6 %, and 0.6 % respectively. RE-LY data is the largest published cardioversion experience to date and the first to evaluate dabigatran in this setting. This reassuring data on dabigatran was regardless of the use of transesophageal echocardiography guidance. Dabigatran is thus a reasonable alternative to warfarin in patients requiring cardioversion. No data are available currently for rivaroxaban and apixaban under these circumstances so that transesophageal echocardiography prior to cardioversion is reasonable in these patients.

AF ablation: AF ablation is associated with a small but definite risk of periprocedural thromboembolic and bleeding complications [77, 78]. The thromboembolic risk can be minimized by adequate periprocedural anticoagulation, which could potentially increase the risk of bleeding. AF ablation on therapeutic warfarin anticoagulation, with an INR of 2 and 3, has been shown to be safe with few thrombotic complications [79–81]. Experience with NOACs in this setting is limited. In observational studies, periprocedural dabigatran was associated with an increased risk of bleeding and composite of bleeding and thromboembolic complications compared with uninterrupted warfarin anticoagulation [81–83]. Patients were however treated with unfractionated heparin (adjusted by in-vitro testing) in combination with the oral therapy so that overlapping pharmacodynamic effect and their relation to the results of in-vitro testing may explain the findings for dabigatran as compared to warfarin. There are currently no controlled data on the risk–benefit profile of catheter ablation on uninterrupted NOACs, thus it is recommended that NOACs should be discontinued before procedure.

Real Life Data

With any new intervention there might be some concern about a potential discrepancy between the safety in clinical trial and real-world clinical experience. Specifically there were lots of concerns raised regarding bleeding risk with NOACs. The clinical trial data support that no increased bleeding liability is associated with the novel oral anticoagulant compared with warfarin; however, reports of serious, and even fatal, bleeding have been published in post-marketing reports.

During 2011 there were 3,781 serious adverse reports related to dabigatran including 542 deaths and at the same time period there were only 1,106 reports related to warfarin (72 deaths). Does this mean that warfarin is safer? The answer is that we can't tell based on this information since it is impossible to judge the magnitude of bias introduced by voluntary reporting when an old drug is compared to a new alternative.

To overcome this limitation the FDA developed the Mini-Sentinel program as part of the Sentinel initiative [84]. The Mini-Sentinel uses pre-existing electronic healthcare data from multiple sources to create an active surveillance system to monitor the safety of FDA-regulated medical products.

In evaluating dabigatran as compared to warfarin the FDA report concentrated on the risk for bleeding in treatment-naive patients. The conclusions were that the actual rates of gastrointestinal hemorrhage and intracranial hemorrhage for new users of dabigatran were lower than bleeding rates associated with new users of warfarin [85]: The combined incidence rate was 1.8–2.6 times higher for new users of warfarin compared with new users of dabigatran. Warfarin use was associated with 1.6–2.2 times higher rate of gastrointestinal hemorrhage risk and 2.1–3.0 times higher rate of intracranial hemorrhage. Like any report based on electronic health care data this report also is not free from unknown confounders but it provides reassurance that dabigatran (and hopefully other NOACs) are at least as safe as warfarin. Similar to any new intervention, it is only long term real world experience that will clarify the exact role of NOACs as antithrombotic agents.

References

1. Camm AJ, Kirchhof P, Lip GY, et al. Guidelines for the management of atrial fibrillation: the task force for the management of atrial fibrillation of the European Society of Cardiology (ESC). Europace. 2010;12:1360–420.
2. De Caterina R, Husted S, Wallentin L, et al. Anticoagulants in heart disease: current status and perspectives. Eur Heart J. 2007;28: 880–913.
3. Camm AJ, Lip GYH, Atar D, et al. 2012 focused update of the ESC guidelines for the management of atrial fibrillation. Eur Heart J. 2012;33:2719–47.

4. Ezekowitz MD, Connolly SJ, Parekh A, et al. Rationale and design of RE-LY: randomized evaluation of long-term anticoagulant therapy, warfarin, compared with dabigatran. Am Heart J. 2009;157: 805–10.

5. Connolly SJ, Ezekowitz MD, Yusuf S, et al. Dabigatran versus warfarin in patients with atrial fibrillation. N Engl J Med. 2009;361:1139–51.

6. Connolly SJ, Ezekowitz MD, Yusuf S, et al. Newly identified events in the RE-LY trial. N Engl J Med. 2010;363:1875–6.

7. Ezekowitz MD, Wallentin L, Connolly SJ, et al.; RE-LY Steering Committee and Investigators. Dabigatran and warfarin in vitamin K antagonist-naive and-experienced cohorts with atrial fibrillation. Circulation 2010;122:2246–53.

8. Patel MR, Mahaffey KW, Garg J, et al. Rivaroxaban versus warfarin in nonvalvular atrial fibrillation. N Engl J Med. 2011;365:883–9.

9. Connolly SJ, Eikelboom J, Joyner C, et al. Apixaban in patients with atrial fibrillation. N Engl J Med. 2011;364:806–17.

10. Granger CB, Alexander JH, McMurray JJ, et al.; ARISTOTLE Committees and Investigators. Apixaban vs. warfarin in patients with atrial fibrillation. N Engl J Med. 2011;365:981–92.

11. ROCKET AF Study Investigators. Rivaroxaban — once daily, oral, direct factor Xa inhibition compared with vitamin K antagonism for prevention of stroke and embolism trial in atrial fibrillation: rationale and design of the ROCKET AF study. Am Heart J. 2010;159:340. e1–7.e1.

12. Lopes RD, Alexander JH, Al-Khatib SM, et al. Apixaban for reduction in stroke and other thromboemboLic events in atrial fibrillation (ARISTOTLE) trial: design and rationale. Am Heart J. 2010;159:331–9.

13. Mueck W, Lensing A, Agnelli G, et al. Rivaroxaban: population pharmacokinetic analyses in patients treated for acute deep-vein thrombosis and exposure simulations in patients with atrial fibrillation treated for stroke prevention. Clin Pharmacokinet. 2011;50:675–86.

14. Weitz JI, Connolly SJ, Patel I, et al. Randomised, parallel-group, multicentre, multinational phase 2 study comparing edoxaban, an oral factor Xa inhibitor, with warfarin for stroke prevention in patients with atrial fibrillation. Thromb Haemost. 2010;104:633–41.

15. Rosendaal FR, Cannegieter SC, van der Meer FJ, Briet E. A method to determine the optimal intensity of oral anticoagulant therapy. Thromb Haemost. 1993;69:236–9.

16. Lip GYH, Larsen TB, Skjøth F, et al. Indirect comparisons of new oral anticoagulant drugs for efficacy and safety when used for stroke prevention in atrial fibrillation. J Am Coll Cardiol. 2012;60:738–46.

17. Dentali F, Riva N, Crowther M, et al. Efficacy and safety of the novel oral anticoagulants in atrial fibrillation: a systematic review and

meta-analysis of the literature. Circulation. 2012;126(20):2381–91 published online October 15, 2012.

18. Weitz JI, Bates SM. New anticoagulants. J Thromb Haemost. 2005;3:1843–53.

19. Smith P, Arnesen H, Holme I. The effect of warfarin on mortality and reinfarction after myocardial infarction. N Engl J Med. 1990;323:1505–11.

20. Hurlen M, Abdelnoor M, Smith P, Erikssen J, Arnesen H. Warfarin, aspirin, or both after myocardial infarction. N Engl J Med. 2002;347:969–74.

21. Lip GY, Huber K, Andreotti F, et al. Management of antithrombotic therapy in atrial fibrillation patients presenting with acute coronary syndrome and/or undergoing percutaneous coronary intervention/stenting. Thromb Haemost. 2010;103:13–28.

22. Faxon DP, Eikelboom JW, Berger PB, et al. Consensus document: antithrombotic therapy in patients with atrial fibrillation undergoing coronary stenting. A North-American perspective. Thromb Haemost. 2011;106:572–84.

23. Connolly S, Pogue J, Hart R, et al. Clopidogrel plus aspirin versus oral anticoagulation for atrial fibrillation in the Atrial fibrillation Clopidogrel Trial with Irbesartan for prevention of Vascular Events (ACTIVE W): a randomised controlled trial. Lancet. 2006;367:1903–12.

24. Hansen ML, Sørensen R, Clausen MT, et al. Risk of bleeding with single, dual, or triple therapy with warfarin, aspirin, and clopidogrel in patients with atrial fibrillation. Arch Intern Med. 2010;170:1433–41.

25. Dewilde WJM, Oirbans T, Verheugt FWA, et al. Use of clopidogrel with or without aspirin in patients taking oral anticoagulant therapy and undergoing percutaneous coronary intervention: an open-label, randomised, controlled trial. Lancet. 2013;381(9872):1107–15.

26. Becker E, Perzborn E, Klipp A, et al. Effects of rivaroxaban ASA and clopidogrel alone and in combination in a porcine model of stent thrombosis. Eur Heart J. 2010;31:904.

27. Mega JL, Braunwald E, Wiviott SD, et al.; for the ATLAS ACS 2-TIMI 51 Investigators. Rivaroxaban in patients with a recent acute coronary syndrome. N Engl J Med. 2012;366:9–19.

28. Dans AL, Connolly SJ, Wallentin L, et al. Concomitant use of antiplatelet therapy with dabigatran or warfarin in the Randomized Evaluation of Long-term Anticoagulation Therapy (RE-LY) trial. Circulation. 2013;127:634–40.

29. Van de Werf F, Brueckman M, Connolly SJ, et al. A comparison of dabigatran etexilate with warfarin in patients with mechanical heart valves: the randomized, phase II study to evaluate the safety and pharmacokinetics of oral dabigatran etexilate in patients after heart valve replacement (RE-ALIGN). Am Heart J. 2012;163:931–7.

30. FDA Drug Safety Communication: Pradaxa (dabigatran etexilate mesylate) should not be used in patients with mechanical prosthetic heart valves. www.fda.gov/Drugs/DrugSafety/ucm332912.htm
31. Weitz JI. New oral anticoagulants: a view from the laboratory. Am J Hematol. 2012;87:S133–6.
32. Orfeo T, Gissel M, Butenas S, et al. Anticoagulants and the propagation phase of thrombin generation. PLoS One. 2011;6:e27852 (Epub ahead of print).
33. Lauer A, Ciancetti FA, Van Cott EM, et al. Anticoagulation with the oral direct thrombin inhibitor dabigatran does not enlarge hematoma volume in experimental intracerebral hemorrhage. Circulation. 2011;124:1654–62.
34. ESC Working Group on Thrombosis. Task force on anticoagulants in heart disease position paper. J Am Coll Cardiol. 2012;59(16):1413–25.
35. Tripodi A. Problems and solutions for testing hemostasis assays whilst patients are on anticoagulants. Semin Thromb Hemost. 2012;38:586–92.
36. Funk DM. Coagulation assays and anticoagulant monitoring. Hematol Am Soc Hematol Educ Program. 2012;2012:460–5.
37. Pradaxa (dabigatran etexilate mesylate) capsules [prescribing information]. Ridgefield: Boehringer Ingelheim Pharmaceuticals, Inc; 2012.
38. van Ryn J, Stangier J, Haertter S, et al. Dabigatran etexilate – a novel, reversible, oral direct thrombin inhibitor: interpretation of coagulation assays and reversal of anticoagulant activity. Thromb Haemost. 2010;103:1116–27.
39. Huisman MV, Lip GY, Diener HC, Brueckmann M, van Ryn J, Clemens A. Dabigatran etexilate for stroke prevention in patients with atrial fibrillation: resolving uncertainties in routine practice. Thromb Haemost. 2012;107:838–47.
40. Eriksson BI, Quinlan DJ, Weitz JI. Comparative pharmacodynamics and pharmacokinetics of oral direct thrombin and factor xa inhibitors in development. Clin Pharmacokinet. 2009;48:1–22.
41. Samama MM, Guinet C. Laboratory assessment of new anticoagulants. Clin Chem Lab Med. 2011;49:761–72.
42. Lindahl TL, Baghaei F, Blixter IF, et al. Effects of the oral, direct thrombin inhibitor dabigatran on five common coagulation assays. Thromb Haemost. 2011;105:371–8.
43. Freyburger G, Macouillard G, Labrouche S, et al. Coagulation parameters in patients receiving dabigatran etexilate or rivaroxaban: two observational studies in patients undergoing total hip or total knee replacement. Thromb Res. 2011;127:457–65.
44. Hillarp A, Baghaei F, Fagerberg IB, et al. Effects of the oral, direct factor Xa inhibitor rivaroxaban on commonly used coagulation assays. J Thromb Haemost. 2011;9:133–9.

45. Mani H, Wagner C, Lindhoff-Last E (2011) Influence of new anticoagulants on coagulation tests. White paper. Siemens Healthcare Diagnostics Inc. www.healthcare.siemens.com/laboratory-diagnostics

46. Stangier J, Feuring M. Using the HEMOCLOT direct thrombin inhibitor assay to determine plasma concentrations of dabigatran. Blood Coagul Fibrinolysis. 2012;23:138–43.

47. Raghavan N, Frost CE, Yu Z, et al. Apixaban metabolism and pharmacokinetics after oral administration to humans. Drug Metab Dispos. 2009;37:74–81.

48. Rohde G. Determination of rivaroxaban – a novel, oral, direct Factor Xa inhibitor – in human plasma by high-performance liquid chromatography-tandem mass spectrometry. J Chromatogr B Analyt Technol Biomed Life Sci. 2008;872:43–50.

49. Van Ryn J, Litzenburger T, Waterman A, et al. Dabigatran anticoagulant activity is neutralized by an antibody selective to dabigatran in in vitro and in vivo models. J Am Coll Cardiol. 2011;57:E1130.

50. Lu G, DeGuzman FR, Lakhotia S, et al. Recombinant antidote for reversal of anticoagulation by factor Xa inhibitors. ASH Annu Meeting Abstr. 2008;112:983.

51. Lu GP, Peng L, Hollenbach SJ, et al. Reconstructed recombinant factor Xa as an antidote to reverse anticoagulation by factor Xa inhibitors. J Thromb Haemost. 2009;7:309.

52. Zhou W, Schwarting S, Illanes S, et al. Hemostatic therapy in experimental intracerebral hemorrhage associated with the direct thrombin inhibitor dabigatran. Stroke. 2011;42:3594–9.

53. Eerenberg ES, Kamphuisen PW, Sijpkens MK, et al. Reversal of rivaroxaban and dabigatran by prothrombin complex concentrate: a randomized, placebo-controlled, crossover study in healthy subjects. Circulation. 2011;124:1573–9.

54. Wolzt M, Levi M, Sarich TC, et al. Effect of recombinant factor VIIa on melagatran-induced inhibition of thrombin generation and platelet activation in healthy volunteers. Thromb Haemost. 2004;91:1090–6.

55. Gruber A, Marzec UM, Buetehorn U, et al. Potential of activated prothrombin complex concentrate and activated factor VII to reverse the anticoagulant effects of rivaroxaban in primates. ASH Annu Meeting Abstr. 2008;112:3825.

56. Escolar G, Arellano-Rodrigo E, Reverter JC, et al. Reversal of apixaban induced alterations of hemostasis by different coagulation factor concentrates: studies in vitro with circulating human blood. Circulation. 2012;126:520–1.

57. Stangier J, Rathgen K, Stahle H, et al. Influence of renal impairment on the pharmacokinetics and pharmacodynamics of oral dabigatran etexilate: an open-label, parallel-group, single-centre study. Clin Pharmacokinet. 2010;49:259–68.

58. Nowak G. The ecarin clotting time, a universal method to quantify direct thrombin inhibitors. Pathophysiol Haemost Thromb. 2003;33:173–83.

59. Barrett YC, Wang Z, Frost C, et al. Clinical laboratory measurement of direct factor Xa inhibitors: anti-Xa assay is preferable to prothrombin time assay. Thromb Haemost. 2010;104:1263–71.

60. Siegal DM, Crowther MA. Acute management of bleeding in patients on novel oral anticoagulants. Eur Heart J. 2013;34:489–98.

61. Kearon C, Hirsh J. Management of anticoagulation before and after elective surgery. N Engl J Med. 1997;336:1506–11.

62. Caliendo FJ, Halpern VJ, Marini CP, et al. Warfarin anticoagulation in the perioperative period: is it safe? Ann Vasc Surg. 1999;13:11–6.

63. Baker WL, Cios DA, Sander SD. Meta-analysis to assess the quality of warfarin control in atrial fibrillation patients in the United States. J Manag Care Pharm. 2009;15:244–52.

64. De Caterina R, Husted S, Wallentin L, et al. New oral anticoagulants in atrial fibrillation and acute coronary syndromes. J Am Coll Cardiol. 2012;59:1413–25.

65. Sie P, Samamab CM, Godier A, et al. Surgery and invasive procedures in patients on long-term treatment with direct oral anticoagulants: thrombin or factor-Xa inhibitors. Recommendations of the working group on perioperative haemostasis and the French study group on thrombosis and haemostasis. Arch Cardiovasc Dis. 2011;104:669–76.

66. Douketis JD. Pharmacologic properties of the new oral anticoagulants: a clinician-oriented review with a focus on perioperative management. Curr Pharm Des. 2010;16:3436–41.

67. Douketis JD, Spyropoulos AC, Spencer FA, et al. Perioperative management of antithrombotic therapy: antithrombotic therapy and prevention of thrombosis, 9th ed.: American College of Chest Physicians Evidence-Based Clinical Practice Guidelines. Chest. 2012;141(2):e326S–50.

68. Douketis JD, Johnson JA, Turpie AG. Low-molecular- weight heparin as bridging anticoagulation during interruption of warfarin: assessment of a standardized periprocedural anticoagulation regimen. Arch Intern Med. 2004;164:1319–26.

69. Alikhan R, et al. The acute management of haemorrhage, surgery and overdose in patients receiving dabigatran. Emerg Med J. 2013;0:1–6. doi:10.1136/emermed-2012-201976.

70. Hankey GJ, Eikelboom JW. Dabigatran etexilate: a new oral thrombin Inhibitor. Circulation. 2011;123:1436–50.

71. Spyropoulos AC, Douketis JD. How I treat anticoagulated patients undergoing an elective procedure or surgery. Blood. 2012;120: 2954–62.

72. Golembiewski J, Chernin E, Chopra T. Prevention and treatment of postoperative nausea and vomiting. Am J Health Syst Pharm. 2005;62:1247–60.

73. Stangier J, Stahle H, Rathgen K, Fuhr R. Pharmacokinetics and pharmacodynamics of the direct oral thrombin inhibitor dabigatran in healthy elderly subjects. Clin Pharmacokinet. 2008;47:47–59.
74. Wanek MR, Horn ET, Elapavaluru S, et al. Safe use of hemodialysis for dabigatran removal before cardiac surgery. Ann Pharmacother. 2012;46:e21.
75. Gogarten W, Vandermeulen E, Van Aken H, et al. Regional anaesthesia and antithrombotic agents: recommendations of the European Society of Anaesthesiology. Eur J Anaesthesiol. 2010;27:999–1015.
76. Nagarakanti R, Ezekowitz MD, Oldgren J, et al. Dabigatran versus warfarin in patients with atrial fibrillation: an analysis of patients undergoing cardioversion. Circulation. 2011;123:131–6.
77. Vazquez SR, Johnson SA, Rondina MT. Peri-procedural anticoagulation in patients undergoing ablation for atrial fibrillation. Thromb Res. 2010;126:e69–77.
78. Viles-Gonzalez JF, Mehta D. Thromboembolic risk and anticoagulation strategies in patients undergoing catheter ablation for atrial fibrillation. Curr Cardiol Rep. 2011;13:38–42.
79. Hakalahti A, Uusimaa P, Ylitalo K. Catheter ablation of atrial fibrillation in patients with therapeutic oral anticoagulation treatment. Europace. 2011;13:640–5.
80. Hussein AA, Martin DO, Saliba W, et al. Radiofrequency ablation of atrial fibrillation under therapeutic international normalized ratio: a safe and efficacious periprocedural anticoagulation strategy. Heart Rhythm. 2009;6:1425–9.
81. Santangeli P, Di Biase L, Sanchez JE. Atrial fibrillation ablation without interruption of anticoagulation. Cardiol Res Pract. 2011;2011:837–41.
82. Spragg DD, Dalal D, Cheema A, et al. Complications of catheter ablation for atrial fibrillation: incidence and predictors. J Cardiovasc Electrophysiol. 2008;19:627–31.
83. Lakkireddy D, Reddy YM, Di Biase L, et al. Feasibility and safety of dabigatran vs. warfarin for periprocedural anticoagulation in patients undergoing radiofrequency ablation for atrial fibrillation results from a multicenter prospective registry. J Am Coll Cardiol. 2012;59:1168–74.
84. Behrman RE, Brenner JS, Brown JS, et al. Developing the sentinel system – a national resource for evidence development. N Engl J Med. 2011;364:498–9.
85. FDA Drug Safety Communication: Update on the risk for serious bleeding events with the anticoagulant Pradaxa (dabigatran). http://www.fda.gov/Drugs/DrugSafety/ucm326580.htm

Chapter 4
Upstream Therapy in the Treatment of Atrial Fibrillation

Cristian Baicus

Introduction

The antiarrhytmic agents, acting as ion channel inhibitors, remain the most important therapy for the rhythm control management of atrial fibrillation (AF), in spite of important advances in nonpharmacological treatment (mainly catheter ablation techniques). However, these treatments are less than optimal when considering efficacy, safety and tolerability [1].

Non-electrical factors, like structural atrial remodelling, probably have an important role in the generation and perpetuation of AF, therefore a therapy which could prevent or even reverse these structural changes might have a place in the primary or secondary prevention of AF. This therapy is called "upstream therapy".

C. Baicus, MD, PhD
Carol Davila University of Medicine and Pharmacy Bucharest, Bucharest, Romania

Department of Internal Medicine,
Colentina University Hospital Bucharest,
Soseaua Stefan cel Mare 19-21, sector 2, 020125,
Bucharest, Romania
e-mail: cbaicus@clicknet.ro

G.-A. Dan et al. (eds.), *Atrial Fibrillation Therapy*, Current Cardiovascular Therapy, DOI 10.1007/978-1-4471-5475-4_4,
© Springer-Verlag London 2014

Rationale and Physiologic Basis

AF is the result of a complex process which consists in both electrical and structural changes of the myocardium, leading to fibrosis and remodelling. Primary prevention should be accomplished by avoiding these changes.

Once appeared, AF itself promotes the continuation of this process of electrical and functional changes, cell death and fibrosis, which self-perpetuates as long as AF persists. Therefore, longer the AF, more important the remodelling, making the reversal to sinus rhythm lesser and lesser possible, therefore the secondary prevention of AF might be possible only with the eventual reversal of these structural modifications.

Targets being parts of the pathways had to be discovered, in order to develop specific therapies, called "upstream". The mechanisms by which upstream therapies may prevent or reduce AF are (a) the prevention of structural remodelling – reduction of fibrosis, inflammation and oxidative stress, (b) the improvement of haemodynamics – lowering left ventricular and left atrial wall stress, and (c) the prevention of coronary artery disease [2].

Both experimental and clinical studies suggested that inflammation, oxidative stress and the renin-angiotensin-aldosterone system (RAAS) play a role in the development of atrial remodelling and fibrosis (Fig. 4.1). While inflammation is involved early, leading to electrical remodelling, RAAS influences both the electrical and structural remodelling from later stages of AF development, being a common pathway of AF regardless of its primary cause [3–5]. Moreover, inflammation stimulates the angiotensin-II production, while angiotensin-II may act as a pro-inflammatory agent in turn. Angiotensin-II has arrhythmogenic effects also by stimulating atrial fibrosis and hypertrophy secondary to activation of mitogen-activated protein kinases, impaired circuit of calcium and activation of oxidative stress mediators [6, 7].

On the other hand, other detrimental effects of RAAS activation are mediated by aldosterone, the incidence of AF

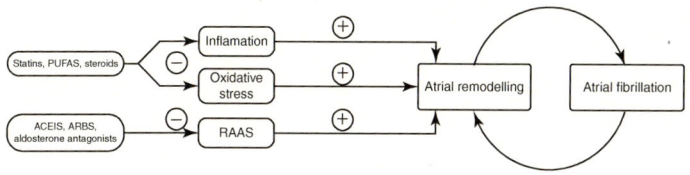

FIGURE 4.1 Physiologic basis of upstream therapy in atrial fibrillation

in patients with primary hyperaldosteronism being 12-fold increased compared to hypertensive controls [8]. Aldosterone might have the same role as angiotensin-II – promoting atrial fibrosis, myocyte hypertrophy, and conduction disturbances, leading again to atrial proarrhythmia imputed directly to aldosterone, since ventricular haemodynamics appeared unaltered in rat models [9].

Inflammation and oxidative stress are also associated with atrial remodelling that promotes AF [3, 10]. The most important arguments are the fact that AF appears after cardiac surgery, during the peak of the inflammatory response, the circulating markers of inflammation are associated with AF, and evidence of oxidative stress was detected in the fibrillating atrium.

A systematic review of case–control studies showed that there might be an association between the angiotensin-converting enzyme insertion/deletion gene polymorphism and atrial fibrillation [11]; however, the odds ratio (OR) was not impressive (1.29), given the potential for bias of case–control studies. Another systematic review found a standardized mean difference of (only) 0.35 units (although statistically significant) in the CRP levels between the patients with, and those without recurrence of AF after successful electrical cardioversion [12].

As a consequence of the above mechanisms, upstream therapies were studied. They would target both the formation and evolution of the substrate for AF. They included angiotensin-converting enzyme inhibitors (ACEIs), angiotensin receptor blockers (ARBs), aldosterone antagonists, statins, and n-3 (v-3) polyunsaturated fatty acids (PUFAs).

The first three block the RAAS, whose role was explained, while statins and PUFAs possess anti-inflammatory and anti-oxidant effects which can counteract inflammatory and oxidative stress pathways which are believed to contribute to the pathogenesis of AF [13].

Concerning upstream therapy, data obtained from experimental studies were judged as "compelling" by some specialists, because most of them, on one hand, supported the mechanisms described above, and on the other hand pleaded for the efficacy of ACEIs, ARBs, aldosterone antagonists, statins, and PUFAs. There were multiple well-conducted experimental studies, and all reported beneficial effects of upstream treatment on electrical and structural remodelling and inducibility of AF [14].

However, experimental evidence is rated only as the fifth level of evidence for clinical practice [15], or is not rated at all [16], as it cannot lead, alone, to clinical recommendations. However, the benchmark research is very important when it leads to new therapeutic ideas which will lately be proven in clinical studies, or the reverse, when it is expected to add to the causality criteria the argument of biological plausibility [17], after epidemiologic studies showed a relationship.

Expectations (From Small Studies) and… Unmet Needs (From RCT)

The problem with the clinical studies concerning upstream therapies is that most of them are observational, retrospective, or post hoc analyses of large randomized trials not primarily designed with AF as a pre-specified endpoint [5].

But they are many, and they were well synthesized in a few reviews, more or less systematic [1, 5, 14, 18, 19]. Every successive review added new studies, as they were published. Of them, the most exhaustive is that of Savelieva [14, 19], which included also a review of the previous meta-analyses.

Concerning the treatment with RAAS blockers and with statins, there are many retrospective and observational studies.

Most of them showed benefits for the RAAS blockers, and mixed results for statins in primary prevention. For the secondary prevention of AF, the open-label studies were positive, while those double-blind, placebo controlled had mixed results.

PUFAs (as fish consumption) were studied mainly in large epidemiologic studies, in which a benefit was associated with higher fish intake for primary prevention, and had mixed results for secondary prevention [14].

Because the risk of AF is higher once the patient had a first episode than before, the number of events is larger in studies concerning the secondary prevention of AF, and the statistical power is higher in these studies, for the same sample of included patients. The same is true for patients after cardiovascular surgery, compared to non-operated patients. Therefore, because of lack of statistical power, there are not small prospective studies specially designed for the primary prevention of AF, excepting those post cardiac surgery with statins. However, there are neither large randomized studies with primary prevention of AF as a primary end-point for any of the upstream therapies.

While the first clinical studies were promising, showing a significant AF reduction with all upstream therapies (ACEIs, ARBs, statins and PUFAs), the results of recent studies – mostly large RCTs (again, not all designed for the AF as endpoint) – were not too optimistic [14, 19–21].

These studies revealed that PUFAs do not significantly reduce the risk of AF (new or recurrent) [14, 19, 22–24], ACEIs and ARBs apparently are effective for primary prevention, but only in patients with systolic heart failure and/or hypertension [22, 25–29]. Statins are clearly effective only in the primary prevention of post-operative AF – there is one RCT on 200 patients (ARMYDA-3), which showed a 61 % relative reduction in the treatment arm, but with a large confidence interval (15–82 %) [30].

Three large randomized controlled studies (RCTs) concerning the secondary prevention of AF with ACEIs and ARBs (GISSI-AF [31], J-RHYTM II [32] and ANTIPAF [33]) did not show any benefit of the treatment – these are the only large RCTs concerning upstream therapies, with AF as primary endpoint. And these studies are most reliable compared to meta-analysis which included other studies without AF as primary endpoint (see below).

Concerning the corticosteroids, the idea that they could decrease the risk of AB by their antinflammatory properties was stressed by some experimental studies. As the inflammation is maximal after cardiac surgery, we might thing that they could have a role to play for the postsurgical AF, like the statins. A systematic review which found seven RCTs on 1,046 patients showed that glucocorticoids significantly reduced the risk of postoperative AF, with an OR of 0.42, and a confidence interval between 0.27 and 0.68 [34]. When the two studies with very high and very low dose of corticosteroids were excluded, the OR was even lower, and the confidence interval narrower, without heterogeneity. Otherwise, there is no evidence to support the use of glucocorticoids for the prevention of AF out of cardiac surgery. On the contrary, epidemiologic studies show that glucocorticoid treatment might be a risk factor for AF [35].

Systematic Reviews with Meta-analyses

We must bear in mind the fact that, although most of them did not include observational studies, these meta-analyses are made of lower quality evidence (almost no RCT with AF as primary endpoint; post-hoc analysis of RCT with other objectives; RCTs with AF followed only as adverse effects), and therefore the meta-analysis themselves cannot be considered high quality evidence.

ACEIs and ARBs

We found more systematic reviews with meta-analysis concerning the treatment with SAAR blockers for the primary [36–38], secondary prevention [39, 40] of AF, or both

[27, 41–44], published from 2004 to 2013 and including between 7,250 and 92,817 patients.

Globally, the treatment reduced the risk of AF fibrillation with between 43 (the smallest and oldest review [36]) and 18 % [37], with relatively large confidence intervals – the lowest margin between 24 [43] and 3 % [37] (relative risk reduction) (Table 4.1). The heterogeneity was important (lowest $I^2 = 75$ %).

If only primary prevention was taken into account, the relative risk reduction was about 20 %, with the lowest margin of the 95 % confidence interval at 7–10 % (Table 4.1).

Concerning the secondary prevention, the risk reduction was more important than in primary prevention (about 50 %), the lowest margin of the confidence interval varying between 11 % and 35 %. A single meta-analysis could not show a reduction of the risk, that of Disertori [39], and consequently the title of his article was: "renin-angiotensin system inhibitors in the prevention of atrial fibrillation recurrences: an unfulfilled hope". The result was close to significance, and probably the meta-analysis lacked enough statistical power, but on the other hand, the largest effects were observed in the smallest studies, and a possible publication bias was revealed by the analysis. And if we take into account the fact that the only large studies which had AF as primary endpoint were negative (see above), probably we could safely conclude that SAAR inhibition does not prevent AF recurrence.

In all meta-analyses, the subgroup analyses showed that the most important effect was present in patients with heart failure, while, surprisingly, the RAAS blockade was not effective at all in patients with hypertension (Table 4.2). There was no effect in patients with coronary disease, diabetes or after myocardial infarction, either [14, 38].

There was no difference between ACEIs and ARBs [38, 44]. Concerning the prevention of AF after coronary artery by-pass grafting, a recent meta-analysis could not draw a conclusion because the studies had conflicting results [45].

Another thing that is worth mentioning is the important heterogeneity of the studies' results, with the lowest I^2 of 75 %.

Table 4.1 Efficacy of RAAS inhibitors in the prevention of AF – meta-analyses (global, primary and secondary prevention)

Publication	Nr patients	Nr studies	RR (95 % CI)
AF, total			
Madrid et al. [36]	24,849	7	0.57 (0.39–0.82)
Healey et al. [27]	56,308	11	0.72 (0.60–0.85)
Anand et al. [37]	69,669	9	0.82 (0.70–0.97)
Jibrini et al. [41]	52,989	11	0.81 (0.76–0.86)
Schneider et al. [42]	87,048	23	0.67 (0.57–0.78)
Zhang et al. [43]	80,524	26	0.65 (0.55–0.76)
Huang et al. [44]	91,381	21	0.75 (0.66–0.85)
Khatib et al. [38]	92,817	14	0.79 (0.69–0.90)
AF, primary prevention			
Madrid et al. [36]	24,849	7	0.57 (0.39–0.82)
Anand et al. [37]	69,669	9	0.82 (0.70–0.97)
Zhang et al. [43]	63,897	8	0.80 (0.70–0.92)
Huang et al. [44]	66,937	9	0.76 (0.65–0.88)
Khatib et al. [38]	92,817	14	0.79 (0.69–0.90)
AF, secondary prevention			
Healey et al. [27]	299	2	0.52 (0.35–0.79)
Jibrini et al. [41]	317	2	0.49 (0.33–0.89)
Schneider et al. [42][a]	1,054	8	0.55 (0.34–0.89)
Schneider et al. [42][b]	1,064	4	0.37 (0.27–0.49)
Zhang et al. [43]	3,260	12	0.45 (0.31–0.65)
Huang et al. [44]	24,444	12	0.73 (0.59–0.89)
Bhuriya et al. [40]	2,323	8	0.61 (0.44–0.85)
Disertori et al. [39][c]	323	4	0.55 (0.38–0.80)
Disertori et al. [39][d]	3,567	5	0.90 (0.75–1.08)

[a]Post cardioversion
[b]Medical therapy studies
[c]ACEIs
[d]ARBs

TABLE 4.2 Efficacy of RAAS inhibitors in the prevention of AF in patients with heart failure and hypertension – meta-analyses

Publication	Nr patients	Nr studies	RR (95 % CI)
Heart failure subgroup			
Healey et al. [27]	10,319	4	0.56 (0.37–0.85)
Anand et al. [37]	11,820	3	0.57 (0.37–0.89)
Jibrini et al. [41]	10,305	4	0.68 (0.59–0.79)
Schneider et al. [42]	11,148	3	0.52 (0.31–0.87)
Zhang et al. [43]	5,972	2	0.60 (0.48–0.75)
Huang et al. [44]	12,294	5	0.58 (0.39–0.87)
Khatib et al. [38]	19,574	5	0.64 (0.48–0.86)
Hypertension subgroup			
Healey et al. [27]	26,403	3	0.88 (0.66–1.19)
Anand et al. [37]	41,324	4	0.94 (0.72–1.23)
Jibrini et al. [41]	26,076	3	0.77 (0.68–0.99)
Schneider et al. [42]	53,494	6	0.89 (0.75–1.05)
Huang et al. [44]	40,421	6	0.71 (0.54–0.92)

The latest meta-analysis [38] searched for the efficacy of aldosterone antagonists, but it failed in finding a proof (2 studies, 8,500 patients, close to statistical significance: highest margin of the confidence interval = 1.08).

Statins

Savelieva [14] commented on six meta-analysis published before 2010, and she concluded that there was no demonstrated value, excepting maybe for patients undergoing cardiac surgery. We identified 18 systematic reviews with meta-analysis published after her review, of which six concerned only AF occurring after cardiac surgery. At the beginning, the meta-analyses included also the observational studies [46–48], and the reduction for the risk of AF was more important. In the same time, the authors identified possible publication bias, and important heterogeneity [46, 49]. Most of the meta-analyses showed a reduction of AF after cardiac surgery [50–52]; strangely, the publication of Yin [48], which included only six observational studies, did not find an effect. Out of surgery, surprisingly, statins appeared more efficient for secondary prevention than for primary prevention [53, 54]. A possible effect was revealed in patients with permanent pacemaker (possibly only in those with sinus node dysfunction) [55] (only 3 studies, 552 patients), or after electrical cardioversion (6 studies, 515 patients, number needed to treat (NNT) = 11) [13]. However, the second largest meta-analysis (32RCTs, 71,000 patients [54]) did not find an effect in primary prevention out of cardiac surgery, while the largest one, which included unpublished data, showed that statins decrease the risk of AF with 39 % only in the analysis of the 13 short time studies, but not in that of the long term studies (22 long term follow-up studies, 105,791 patients [49]). A recent Cochrane review concluded that preoperative statin therapy reduces the odds of post-operative AF, but since the analyzed studies included mainly patients undergoing myocardial revascularizations, the results cannot be extrapolated to patients undergoing other cardiac procedures such as heart valve or aortic surgery [56].

PUFAs

We found six systematic reviews with meta-analysis concerning the effect with PUFAs in the prevention of AF, published between 2011 and 2013. One of them [57] included observational studies, too, while the other, which included only RCTs, analyzed relatively small samples (the largest had 1,900 patients). An important heterogeneity was present.

Two meta-analyses were dedicated to secondary prevention [58, 59], one investigated the primary prevention [60], one investigated both, while two were interested in postoperative AF [61, 62].

No meta-analysis showed an effect of PUFAs in reducing the risk of new onset or recurrent AF, after cardiac surgery or not.

Guidelines

The American College of Cardiology/American Heart Association/European Society of Cardiology guidelines from 2006 [63] decided that the role for upstream therapy needed further clarification before recommendations could be made, and no reference to upstream therapy was made in the updated version of the guideline [64].

The European Society of Cardiology AF guidelines from 2010 [65] recommended ACEIs and ARBs for the new onset atrial fibrillation in patients with heart failure and reduced ejection fraction (weak recommendation, ESC class IIa, level A) and for those with hypertension, particularly left ventricular hypertrophy (ESC Class IIa, Level B), and it did not recommend it in patients without cardiovascular disease. Statins were recommended to be considered for the prevention of AF after coronary artery bypass grafting, isolated or in combination with valvular interventions (ESC class IIa, level B) and were not recommended for the prevention of AF in patients without cardiovascular disease (ESC class IIb, level B). Therefore, these drugs were indicated in instances in which they were already prescribed (ACEIs and ARBs in systolic heart failure and hypertension, statins in coronary artery disease).

However, the 2012 update of the guidelines [66] took into account the fact that the recent RCTs with ARBs and the majority with those with PUFAs "failed to show convincing results", and therefore there is little reason to recommend these therapies for the prevention of AF recurrence in patients with little or no underlying heart disease, but it might be justified to add an ACEI or ARB to an antiarrhythmic drug after cardioversion.

In conclusion, the clinical studies show that upstream therapy might be efficient in primary AF prevention, delaying

102   C. Baicus

atrial structural remodelling, but probably it cannot reverse it if already established. The recent studies of upstream therapy have been negative, but additional investigations are needed to search into the potential effect of specific upstream therapy agents in specific AF pathologies, focusing on early stages of atrial structural remodelling [1].

References

1. Burashnikov A, Antzelevitch C. Novel pharmacological targets for the rhythm control management of atrial fibrillation. Pharmacol Ther. 2011;132(3):300–13.
2. Van Gelder IC. Rhythm control for atrial fibrillation: non-channel antiarrhythmic drugs are en vogue. Cardiovasc Res. 2007;74:8–10.
3. Murray KT, Mace LC, Yang Z. Non-antiarrhythmic drug therapy for atrial fibrillation. Heart Rhythm. 2007;4:S88–90.
4. Ehrlich JR, Hohnloser SH, Nattel S. Role of angiotensin system and effects of its inhibition in atrial fibrillation: clinical and experimental evidence. Eur Heart J. 2006;27:512–8.
5. Dorian P, Singh BN. Upstream therapies to prevent AF. Eur Heart J Suppl. 2008;10:H11–31.
6. Goette A, Lendeckel U. Electrophysiological effects of angiotensin II. Part I: signal transduction and basic electrophysiological mechanisms. Europace. 2008;10:238–41.
7. Cardin S, Li D, Thorin-Trescases N, Leung TK, Thorin E, Nattel S. Evolution of the atrial fibrillation substrate in experimental congestive heart failure: angiotensin-dependent and -independent pathways. Cardiovasc Res. 2003;60:315–25.
8. Milliez P, Girerd X, Plouin PF, Blacher J, Safar ME, Mourad JJ. Evidence for an increased rate of cardiovascular events in patients with primary aldosteronism. J Am Coll Cardiol. 2005;45:1243–8.
9. Reil JC, Hohl M, Selejan S, Lipp P, Drautz F, Kazakow A, et al. Aldosterone promotes atrial fibrillation. Eur Heart J. 2012;33: 2098–108.
10. Burstein B, Nattel S. Atrial structural remodeling as an antiarrhythmic target. J Cardiovasc Pharmacol. 2008;52:4–10.
11. Liu T, Korantzopoulos P, Xu G, Shehata M, Li D, Wang Z, et al. Association between angiotensin-converting enzyme insertion/deletion gene polymorphism and atrial fibrillation: a meta-analysis. Europace. 2011;13:346–54.
12. Liu T, Li L, Korantzopoulos P, Goudevenos JA, Li G. Association between C-reactive protein and recurrence of atrial fibrillation after

successful electrical cardioversion: a meta-analysis. J Am Coll Cardiol. 2007;49:1642–8.

13. Loffredo L, Angelico F, Perri L, Violi F. Upstream therapy with statin and recurrence of atrial fibrillation after electrical cardioversion. Review of the literature and meta-analysis. BMC Cardiovasc Disord. 2012;12:107.

14. Savelieva I, Kakouros N, Kourliouros A, Camm AJ. Upstream therapies for management of atrial fibrillation: review of clinical evidence and implications for European Society of Cardiology guidelines. Part I: primary prevention. Europace. 2011;13:308–28.

15. OCEBM Levels of Evidence Working Group. The Oxford 2011 levels of evidence. Oxford Centre for Evidence-Based Medicine. http://www.cebm.net/index.aspx?o=5653. Accessed 25 July 2013.

16. Guyatt GH, Oxman AD, Vist GE, Kunz R, Falck-Ytter Y, Alonso-Coello P, Schünemann HJ, for the GRADE Working Group. GRADE: an emerging consensus on rating quality of evidence and strength of recommendations. BMJ. 2008;336:924–6.

17. Hill AB. The environment and disease: association or causation? Proc R Soc Med. 1965;58:295–300.

18. Smit MD, Van Gelder IC. Upstream therapy of atrial fibrillation. Expert Rev Cardiovasc Ther. 2009;7:763–78.

19. Savelieva I, Kakouros N, Kourliouros A, Camm AJ. Upstream therapies for management of atrial fibrillation: review of clinical evidence and implications for European society of cardiology guidelines. Part II: secondary prevention. Europace. 2011;13:610–25.

20. Almroth H, Hoglund N, Boman K, Englund A, Jensen S, Kjellman B, et al. Atorvastatin and persistent atrial fibrillation following cardioversion: a randomized placebo-controlled multicentre study. Eur Heart J. 2009;30:827–33.

21. Schwartz GG, Chaitman BR, Goldberger JJ, Messig M. High-dose atorvastatin and risk of atrial fibrillation in patients with prior stroke or transient ischemic attack: analysis of the Stroke Prevention by Aggressive Reduction in Cholesterol Levels (SPARCL) trial. Am Heart J. 2011;161:993–9.

22. Camm AJ, Kirchhof P, Lip GY, Schotten U, Savelieva I, Ernst S, et al. Guidelines for the management of atrial fibrillation: the task force for the management of atrial fibrillation of the European Society of Cardiology (ESC). Eur Heart J. 2010;12:1360–420.

23. Kowey PR, Reiffel JA, Ellenbogen KA, Naccarelli GV, Pratt CM. Efficacy and safety of prescription omega-3 fatty acids for the prevention of recurrent symptomatic atrial fibrillation: a randomized controlled trial. JAMA. 2010;304:2363–72.

24. Bianconi L, Calo L, Mennuni M, Santini L, Morosetti P, Azzolini P, et al. n-3 Polyunsaturated fatty acids for the prevention of arrhythmia recurrence after electrical cardioversion of chronic persistent atrial fibrillation: a randomized, double-blind, multicentre study. Europace. 2011;13:174–81.

25. Disertori M, Latini R, Barlera S, Franzosi MG, Staszewsky L, Maggioni AP, et al. Valsartan for prevention of recurrent atrial fibrillation. N Engl J Med. 2009;360:1606–17.
26. Yusuf S, Healey JS, Pogue J, Chrolavicius S, Flather M, Hart RG, et al. Irbesartan in patients with atrial fibrillation. N Engl J Med. 2011;364:928–38.
27. Healey JS, Baranchuk A, Crystal E, Morillo CA, Garfinkle M, Yusuf S, et al. Prevention of atrial fibrillation with angiotensin-converting enzyme inhibitors and angiotensin receptor blockers: a meta-analysis. J Am Coll Cardiol. 2005;45:1832–9.
28. Maggioni AP, Fabbri G, Lucci D, Marchioli R, Franzosi MG, Latini R, et al. Effects of rosuvastatin on atrial fibrillation occurrence: ancillary results of the GISSI-HF trial. Eur Heart J. 2009;30: 2327–36.
29. Ducharme A, Swedberg K, Pfeffer MA, Cohen-Solal A, Granger CB, Maggioni AP, et al. Prevention of atrial fibrillation in patients with symptomatic chronic heart failure by candesartan in the Candesartan in Heart failure: Assessment of Reduction in Mortality and morbidity (CHARM) program. Am Heart J. 2006;152:86–92.
30. Patti G, Chello M, Candura D, Pasceri V, D'Ambrosio A, Covino E, et al. Randomized trial of atorvastatin for reduction of postoperative atrial fibrillation in patients undergoing cardiac surgery: results of the ARMYDA-3 (Atorvastatin for Reduction of MYocardial Dysrhythmia After cardiac surgery) study. Circulation. 2006;114:1455–61.
31. GISSI-AF Investigators, Disertori M, Latini R, Barlera S, Franzosi MG, Staszewsky L, Maggioni AP, et al. Valsartan for prevention of recurrent atrial fibrillation. N Engl J Med. 2009;360:1606–17.
32. Yamashita T, Inoue H, Okumura K, Kodama I, Aizawa Y, Atarashi H, et al.; J-RHYTHM II Investigators. Randomized trial of angiotensin II-receptor blocker vs. dihydropiridine calcium channel blocker in the treatment of paroxysmal atrial fibrillation with hypertension (J-RHYTHM II study). Europace. 2011;13:473–9.
33. Goette A, Schön N, Kirchhof P, Breithardt G, Fetsch T, Häusler KG, et al. Angiotensin II-antagonist in paroxysmal atrial fibrillation (ANTIPAF) trial. Circ Arrhythm Electrophysiol. 2012;5:43–51.
34. Marik PE, Fromm R. The efficacy and dosage effect of corticosteroids for the prevention of atrial fibrillation after cardiac surgery: a systematic review. J Crit Care. 2009;24:458–63.
35. Christiansen CF, Christensen S, Mehnert F, Cummings SR, Chapurlat RD, Sørensen HT. Glucocorticoid use and risk of atrial fibrillation or flutter: a population-based, case–control study. Arch Intern Med. 2009;169:1677–83.
36. Madrid AH, Peng J, Zamora J, Marín I, Bernal E, Escobar C, et al. The role of angiotensin receptor blockers and/or angiotensin converting enzyme inhibitors in the prevention of atrial fibrillation in

patients with cardiovascular diseases: meta-analysis of randomized controlled clinical trials. Pacing Clin Electrophysiol. 2004;27: 1405–10.

37. Anand K, Mooss AN, Hee TT, Mohiuddin SM. Meta-analysis: inhibition of renin-angiotensin system prevents new-onset atrial fibrillation. Am Heart J. 2006;152:217–22.

38. Khatib R, Joseph P, Briel M, Yusuf S, Healey J. Blockade of the renin-angiotensin-aldosterone system (RAAS) for primary prevention of non-valvular atrial fibrillation: a systematic review and meta analysis of randomized controlled trials. Int J Cardiol. 2013;165:17–24.

39. Disertori M, Barlera S, Staszewsky L, Latini R, Quintarelli S, Franzosi MG. Systematic review and meta-analysis: renin-angiotensin system inhibitors in the prevention of atrial fibrillation recurrences: an unfulfilled hope. Cardiovasc Drugs Ther. 2012;26:47–54.

40. Bhuriya R, Singh M, Sethi A, Molnar J, Bahekar A, Singh PP, et al. Prevention of recurrent atrial fibrillation with angiotensin-converting enzyme inhibitors or angiotensin receptor blockers: a systematic review and meta-analysis of randomized trials. J Cardiovasc Pharmacol Ther. 2011;16:178–84.

41. Jibrini MB, Molnar J, Arora RR. Prevention of atrial fibrillation by way of abrogation of the renin-angiotensin system: a systematic review and meta-analysis. Am J Ther. 2008;15:36–43.

42. Schneider MP, Hua TA, Bohm M, Wachtell K, Kjeldsen SE, Schmieder RE. Prevention of atrial fibrillation by renin-angiotensin system inhibition a meta-analysis. J Am Coll Cardiol. 2010;55: 2299–307.

43. Zhang Y, Zhang P, Mu Y, Gao M, Wang JR, Wang Y, et al. The role of renin-angiotensin system blockade therapy in the prevention of atrial fibrillation: a meta-analysis of randomized controlled trials. Clin Pharmacol Ther. 2010;88(4):521–31.

44. Huang G, Xu JB, Liu JX, He Y, Nie XL, Li Q, et al. Angiotensin-converting enzyme inhibitors and angiotensin receptor blockers decrease the incidence of atrial fibrillation: a meta-analysis. Eur J Clin Invest. 2011;41:719–33.

45. Johnston K, Stephens S. Effect of angiotensin-converting enzyme inhibitors and angiotensin receptor blockers on risk of atrial fibrillation before coronary artery bypass grafting. Ann Pharmacother. 2012;46:1239–44.

46. Liakopoulos OJ, Choi YH, Kuhn EW, Wittwer T, Borys M, Madershahian N, et al. Statins for prevention of atrial fibrillation after cardiac surgery: a systematic literature review. J Thorac Cardiovasc Surg. 2009;138:678–86.

47. Saso S, Vecht JA, Rao C, Protopapas A, Ashrafian H, Leff D, et al. Statin therapy may influence the incidence of postoperative atrial fibrillation: what is the evidence? Tex Heart Inst J. 2009;36:521–9.

48. Yin L, Wang Z, Wang Y, Ji G, Xu Z. Effect of statins in preventing postoperative atrial fibrillation following cardiac surgery. Heart Lung Circ. 2010;19:579–83.
49. Rahimi K, Emberson J, McGale P, Majoni W, Merhi A, Asselbergs FW, et al.; PROSPER Executive. Effect of statins on atrial fibrillation: collaborative meta-analysis of published and unpublished evidence from randomised controlled trials. BMJ. 2011;342:d1250.
50. Chen WT, Krishnan GM, Sood N, Kluger J, Coleman CI. Effect of statins on atrial fibrillation after cardiac surgery: a duration- and dose–response meta-analysis. J Thorac Cardiovasc Surg. 2010;140(2):364–72.
51. Winchester DE, Wen X, Xie L, Bavry AA. Evidence of pre-procedural statin therapy a meta-analysis of randomized trials. J Am Coll Cardiol. 2010;56:1099–109.
52. Dong L, Zhang F, Shu X. Usefulness of statins pretreatment for the prevention of postoperative atrial fibrillation in patients undergoing cardiac surgery. Ann Med. 2011;43:69–74.
53. Fang WT, Li HJ, Zhang H, Jiang S. The role of statin therapy in the prevention of atrial fibrillation: a meta-analysis of randomized controlled trials. Br J Clin Pharmacol. 2012;74:744–56.
54. Fauchier L, Clementy N, Babuty D. Statin therapy and atrial fibrillation: systematic review and updated meta-analysis of published randomized controlled trials. Curr Opin Cardiol. 2013;28(1):7–18.
55. Santangeli P, Ferrante G, Pelargonio G, Dello Russo A, Casella M, Bartoletti S, et al. Usefulness of statins in preventing atrial fibrillation in patients with permanent pacemaker: a systematic review. Europace. 2010;12:649–54.
56. Liakopoulos OJ, Kuhn EW, Slottosch I, Wassmer G, Wahlers T. Preoperative statin therapy for patients undergoing cardiac surgery. Cochrane Database Syst Rev. 2012;4:CD008493.
57. Khawaja O, Gaziano JM, Djoussé L. A meta-analysis of omega-3 fatty acids and incidence of atrial fibrillation. J Am Coll Nutr. 2012;31:4–13.
58. Cao H, Wang X, Huang H, Ying SZ, Gu YW, Wang T, et al. Omega-3 fatty acids in the prevention of atrial fibrillation recurrences after cardioversion: a meta-analysis of randomized controlled trials. Intern Med. 2012;51:2503–8.
59. He Z, Yang L, Tian J, Yang K, Wu J, Yao Y. Efficacy and safety of omega-3 fatty acids for the prevention of atrial fibrillation: a meta-analysis. Can J Cardiol. 2013;29:196–203.
60. Liu T, Korantzopoulos P, Shehata M, Li G, Wang X, Kaul S. Prevention of atrial fibrillation with omega-3 fatty acids: a meta-analysis of randomised clinical trials. Heart. 2011;97:1034–40.
61. Armaganijan L, Lopes RD, Healey JS, Piccini JP, Nair GM, Morillo CA. Do omega-3 fatty acids prevent atrial fibrillation after open

heart surgery? A meta-analysis of randomized controlled trials. Clinics (Sao Paulo). 2011;66:1923–8.

62. Benedetto U, Angeloni E, Melina G, Danesi TH, Di Bartolomeo R, Lechiancole A, et al. n-3 Polyunsaturated fatty acids for the prevention of postoperative atrial fibrillation: a meta-analysis of randomized controlled trials. J Cardiovasc Med (Hagerstown). 2013;14:104–9.

63. Fuster V, Rydén LE, Cannom DS, Crijns HJ, Curtis AB, Ellenbogen KA, et al.; American College of Cardiology/American Heart Association Task Force on Practice Guidelines; European Society of Cardiology Committee for Practice Guidelines; European Heart Rhythm Association; Heart Rhythm Society. ACC/AHA/ESC 2006 guidelines for the management of patients with atrial fibrillation: a report of the American College of Cardiology/American Heart Association Task Force on Practice Guidelines and the European Society of Cardiology Committee for Practice Guidelines (Writing Committee to Revise the 2001 guidelines for the management of patients with atrial fibrillation): developed in collaboration with the European Heart Rhythm Association and the Heart Rhythm Society. Circulation. 2006;114:e257–354.

64. American College of Cardiology Foundation, American Heart Association, European Society of Cardiology, Heart Rhythm Society, Wann LS, Curtis AB, Ellenbogen KA, Estes NA, Ezekowitz MD, Jackman WM, et al. Management of patients with atrial fibrillation (compilation of 2006 ACCF/AHA/ESC and 2011 ACCF/AHA/HRS recommendations): a report of the American College of Cardiology/American Heart Association Task Force on practice guidelines. Circulation. 2013;127:1916–26.

65. Camm AJ, Kirchhof P, Lip GY, Schotten U, Savelieva I, Ernst S, et al.; European Heart Rhythm Association, European Association for Cardio-Thoracic Surgery. Guidelines for the management of atrial fibrillation: the Task Force for the Management of Atrial Fibrillation of the European Society of Cardiology (ESC). Eur Heart J. 2010;31:2369–429.

66. Camm AJ, Lip GY, De Caterina R, Savelieva I, Atar D, Hohnloser SH, et al. 2012 focused update of the ESC Guidelines for the management of atrial fibrillation: an update of the 2010 ESC Guidelines for the management of atrial fibrillation. Developed with the special contribution of the European Heart Rhythm Association. Eur Heart J. 2012;33:2719–47.

Chapter 5
Drug Therapy for Rhythm and Rate Control in Atrial Fibrillation

Josep Guindo Soldevila and Antoni Martinez-Rubio

Atrial fibrillation (AF) is the most common sustained cardiac arrhythmia in clinical practice. It is not a benign disease because is associated to a significant increase in mortality and morbidity. Thus, because AF is a potentially dangerous arrhythmia, it seems logical to use antiarrhythmic strategies to avoid, or at least control, this rhythm disturbance [1, 2].

Pharmacologic Rate Control Versus Rhythm Control

There are two main strategies to manage AF: rhythm control (restoration followed by maintenance of sinus rhythm with either antiarrhythmic drugs or radiofrequency catheter ablation); and rate control with atrioventricular (AV) nodal modulators.

J.G. Soldevila, MD (✉)
Cardiology Service, Hospital Parc Tauli de Sabadell,
Sabadell, Barcelona, Spain
e-mail: josepguindo@gmail.com

A. Martinez-Rubio, MD, PhD, MsHM, FESC, FACC
Department of Cardiology, University Hospital
of Sabadell, Sabadell, Barcelona, Spain

G.-A. Dan et al. (eds.), *Atrial Fibrillation Therapy*, Current Cardiovascular Therapy, DOI 10.1007/978-1-4471-5475-4_5, © Springer-Verlag London 2014

The main reason to initiate rhythm control therapy is relief of AF-related symptoms. Conversely, asymptomatic patients (or those who become asymptomatic with adequate rate control therapy) should not generally receive antiarrhythmic drugs. There is no definitive evidence that one strategy is superior to the other. The choice between a rhythm- or a rate-control strategy should be determined by many factors, including the nature, frequency, and severity of symptoms, the length of time that AF has been present continuously in patients with persistent AF, left atrial size, comorbidities, the response to prior cardioversions, age, the side effects and efficacy of the antiarrhythmic drugs already used to treat the patient, and the patient's preference.

Several randomized studies have compared a rate-control strategy with a rhythm-control strategy in patients with AF. The AFFIRM study [3], was the largest study, including 4,060 patients. At 5 years of follow-up, the prevalence of sinus rhythm was 35 % in the rate-control arm and 63 % in the rhythm-control arm. However, there was no significant difference between the two study arms in total mortality, stroke rate, or quality of life. The percentage of patients requiring hospitalization was significantly lower in the rate-control arm (73 %) than in the rhythm-control arm (80 %), and the incidence of adverse drug effects such as torsades de pointes also was significantly lower in the rate-control arm (0.2 % vs. 0.8 %). The authors of the AFFIRM study concluded that there is no survival advantage of a rhythm-control strategy over a rate-control strategy and that a rate-control strategy has advantages such as a lower probability of hospitalization and of drug adverse effects. In a post-hoc analysis [4] sinus rhythm was found to be independently associated with lower mortality (hazard ratio, 0.53), and antiarrhythmic drug therapy was independently associated with increased mortality (hazard ratio, 1.49). Therefore, the potential benefit of maintaining sinus rhythm with antiarrhythmic drugs was negated by the adverse effects of the antiarrhythmic drug therapy.

More recently, Tsadok et al. [5] analyzed prescription and follow-up data of 57,518 patients with AF. They reported that in comparison with rate control therapy (n = 41,193), the use of rhythm control therapy (n = 16,325) was associated with lower rates of stroke/transient ischemic attack (TIA), in particular, among those patients with moderate and high risk of stroke. The crude stroke/TIA incidence rate was 1.74 versus 2.49, per 100 person-years (p < 0.001), respectively. This observation was documented although treatment with any antithrombotic drug was comparable in the two groups (76.8 % in rhythm control vs. 77.8 % in rate control group).

Pharmacologic Therapy for Rhythm Control

Drug therapy for rhythm control in patients with AF may be used in two different clinical scenarios:

- Pharmacological cardioversion.
- Long-term antiarrhythmic drugs to maintain sinus rhythm

Pharmacological Cardioversion

Although acute AF frequently terminates spontaneously within the first hours or days, pharmacological cardioversion may be necessary in some patients. The conversion rate with antiarrhythmic drugs is lower than with direct current cardioversion, but does not require conscious sedation or anaesthesia, and may facilitate the choice of antiarrhythmic drug therapy to prevent new episodes of AF. It is important to note, however, that continuous medical supervision and ECG monitoring is mandatory during drug therapy to detect proarrhythmic events (ventricular proarrhythmia, sinus node arrest, or atrioventricular block).

Several agents are available for pharmacological cardioversion (Table 5.1).

Flecainide given i.v. (usual dose is 2 mg/kg over 10 min) is highly effective for restoring sinus rhythm (67–92 % at 6 h) on restoring sinus rhythm. Oral administration of flecainide

TABLE 5.1 Drugs and doses for pharmacological conversion of recent-onset AF [2]

Drug	Dose	Precautions
Amiodarone	5 mg/kg i.v. over 1 h; 50 mg/h	Phlebitis, hypotension
Flecainide	2 mg/kg i.v. over 10 min, or 200–300 mg p.o	Contraindicated in patients with structural heart disease; may prolong QRS duration and QT Interval. May increase ventricular rate due to conversion to atrial flutter and 1:1 conduction to the ventricles
Ibutilide	1 mg i.v. over 10 min; 1 mg i.v. over 10 min after waiting for 10 min	May prolong QT interval and cause torsades de pointes
Propafenone	2 mg/kg i.v. over 10 min, or 450–600 mg p.o	Contraindicated in patients with structural heart disease; may prolong QRS duration; May increase ventricular rate due to conversion to atrial flutter and 1:1 conduction to the ventricles
Vernakalant	3 mg/kg i.v. over 10 min; second infusion of 2 mg/kg i.v. over 10 min after 15 min rest	Contraindicated in patients with systolic blood pressure <100 mmHg, severe aortic stenosis, heart failure (class NYHA III and IV), acute coronary syndrome within the previous 30 days, or QT interval prolongation

(200–400 mg) may also be effective for recent onset AF. Flecainide should be avoided in patients with underlying heart disease, particularly ischemic heart disease and left ventricular dysfunction.

Intravenous *propafenone* (2 mg/kg over 10–20 min) has a conversion rate between 41 % and 91 %. Propafenone may also be effective after oral administration (450–600 mg). Similar to flecainide, propafenone should be avoided in patients with underlying heart disease.

Intravenous *amiodarone* (5 mg/kg over 1 h; perfusion 50 mg/h) is also effective but cardioversion occurs several hours later than with flecainide or propafenone. The approximate conversion rate at 24 h in placebo-treated patients was 40–60 %, with an increase to 80–90 % after amiodarone treatment. The main side effects of i.v. amiodarone are hypotension (mainly associated with a fast bolus) and phlebitis.

Ibutilide given i.v. (one or two infusions of 1 mg over 10 min each, with a wait of 10 min between doses), has demonstrated the faster cardioversion rates in patients with recent-onset AF. After Ibutilide i.v administration the conversion rates within 90 min is about 50 %. Ibutilide is even more effective for conversion of atrial flutter than AF. The most important side effects are QT interval prolongation and polymorphic ventricular tachycardia. The QTc interval is expected to increase by approximately 60 ms. Therefore, this drug is not used in several countries.

Vernakalant (3 mg/kg i.v. over 10 min, followed if necessary by a second infusion of 2 mg/kg over 10 min after 15 min) has been recently approved for pharmacological cardioversion of AF. In the AVRO Trial (Phase III prospective, randomized, double-blind, Active-controlled, multi-center, superiority study of Vernakalant injection versus amiodarone in subjects with Recent Onset atrial fibrillation) [6], Vernakalant was more effective than amiodarone for the rapid conversion of AF to sinus rhythm (51.7 % vs. 5.7 % at 90 min after the start of treatment; P < 0.0001) [6]. Vernakalant is contraindicated in patients with systolic blood pressure <100 mmHg, severe aortic stenosis, heart failure (class NYHA III and IV), acute coronary syndrome within the previous 30 days, or QT interval prolongation. Before its use, the patients should be adequately hydrated. ECG and hemodynamic monitoring should be used, and the infusion can be followed by direct current cardioversion if necessary. This drug is not contraindicated in patients with stable coronary artery disease, hypertensive heart disease, or mild heart failure.

The experience with other drugs (digoxin, verapamil, beta-blockers, sotalol) in acute AF cardioversion is scarce or ineffective.

In summary, following the recommendation of the European Society of Cardiology (ESC) Guidelines [2] in suitable patients with recent-onset AF (generally 48 h duration), an attempt to pharmacological cardioversion to sinus rhythm can be offered with i.v. flecainide or propafenone (when there is little or no underlying structural heart disease) or amiodarone (when there is structural disease). The anticipated conversion rate is $\geq$50 % within 15–120 min. Ibutilide is effective, but the risk of serious proarrhythmia is not negligible.

Long-term Antiarrhythmic Drugs to Maintain Sinus Rhythm

As explained before, there is no evidence that the pharmacological rhythm control strategy is superior to rate control. Accordingly with the ESC Guidelines [2], the principles of antiarrhythmic drug therapy to maintain sinus rhythm in AF are:

1. Treatment is motivated by attempts to reduce AF-related symptoms.
2. Efficacy of antiarrhythmic drugs to maintain sinus rhythm is only modest.
3. Clinically successful antiarrhythmic drug therapy may reduce rather than eliminate recurrence of AF.
4. If one antiarrhythmic drug 'fails', a clinically acceptable response may be achieved with another agent.
5. Drug-induced proarrhythmia or extra-cardiac side effects are frequent.
6. Safety rather than efficacy considerations should primarily guide the choice of antiarrhythmic agent

In Cochrane Database meta-analysis including 44 randomized controlled trials comparing antiarrhythmic drugs (disopyramide, quinidine, flecainide, propafenone, dofetilide, sotalol, amiodarone) against control (placebo or no treatment), demonstrated that antiarrhythmic drugs significantly reduced the rate of recurrent AF [7]. The likelihood of maintaining sinus rhythm is approximately doubled by the use of antiarrhythmic drugs. Amiodarone was superior to class I agents and sotalol.

Beta-Blockers are only modestly effective in preventing recurrent AF, except in the context of thyrotoxicosis and exercise-induced AF. In a randomized trial in 394 patients, patients receiving metoprolol had a 47.7 % AF relapse rate compared with 59.9 % in controls (P = 0.005).

The most currently used antiarrhythmic drugs for preventing recurrences and maintaining sinus rhythm in AF patients are flecainide, propafenone, sotalol, amiodarone and dronedarone (Table 5.2). *Quinidine* was one of the first antiarrhythmic drugs used for maintenance of sinus rhythm in patients with AF. However, its use is now largely abandoned because the results of a meta-analysis demonstrating that quinidine increased mortality, very probably due to ventricular proarrhythmia secondary to QT interval prolongation (torsade de pointes). *Disopyramide* is only reserved for some cases of vagally induced AF.

Flecainide (100–200 mg b.i.d) is one of the most effective antiarrhythmic drugs for preventing AF recurrences. It can be safely administered in patients without significant structural heart disease, but is contraindicated in patients with more than moderate renal failure (creatinine clearance <50 mg/mL), coronary artery disease, or reduced LVEF. Caution should be observed in the presence of intraventricular conduction delay (particularly left bundle branch block). During flecainide therapy (upon initiation or after a dose increase), regular ECG monitoring is mandatory; an increase in QRS duration of >25 % during flecainide therapy is a sign of potential risk of proarrhythmia and the drug should be stopped or the dose reduced. On the other hand, it should be remembered that during AF relapses, flecainide may facilitate the conversion of AF to atrial flutter, which then may be conducted rapidly to the ventricles. For this reason concomitant atrioventricular node blockade is recommended in patients receiving flecainide (or propafenone).

Propafenone (150–300 mg/t.i.d) prevents recurrent AF in a same way as flecainide. Propafenone has a weak

TABLE 5.2 Antiarrhythmic drugs most commonly used in control rhythm of patients with AF [2]

Drug	Dose	Precautions
Disopyramide	100–250 mg t.i.d	Contraindicated in systolic heart failure
		Caution when using concomitant therapy with QT-prolonging drugs. Lower dose/discontinuation if QT interval >500 ms
Flecainide	100–200 mg b.i.d	Contraindicated if creatinine clearance <50 mg/mL, in coronary artery disease, reduced LV ejection fraction. Caution in the presence of conduction system disease. Lower dose/discontinuation if QRS duration increase >25 % above baseline
Propafenone	150–300 mg t.i.d	Contraindicated in coronary artery disease, reduced LV ejection fraction. Caution in the presence of conduction system disease and renal impairment. Lower dose/discontinuation if QRS duration increase >25 % above baseline
d,l-Sotalol	80–160 mg b.i.d	Contraindicated in the presence of significant LV hypertrophy, systolic heart failure, pre-existing QT prolongation, hypokalaemia, creatinine clearance <50 mg/mL. Moderate renal dysfunction requires careful adaptation of dose. May slow AV conduction (similar to high-dose of beta-blockers). Lower dose/discontinuation if QT interval >500 ms

(continued)

TABLE 5.2 (continued)

Drug	Dose	Precautions
Amiodarone	600 mg o.d. for 4 weeks, 400 mg o.d. for 4 weeks, then 200 mg o.d	Caution when using concomitant therapy with QT-prolonging drugs, heart failure. Dose of vitamin K antagonists and of digitoxin/digoxin should be reduced. . Lower dose/discontinuation if QT interval >500 ms
Dronedarone	400 mg b.i.d	Contraindicated in NYHA class III–IV or unstable heart failure, during concomitant therapy with QT-prolonging drugs, powerful CYP3A4 inhibitors, and creatinine clearance <30 mg/mL. Caution when using concomitant therapy with QT-prolonging drugs, heart failure. Dose of digitoxin/digoxin should be reduced. Elevations in serum creatinine of 0.1–0.2 mg/dL are common and do not reflect reduced renal function. . Lower dose/discontinuation if QT interval >500 ms

beta-adrenoreceptor blocking effect. It can be safely administered in patients without significant structural heart disease, but should not be used in patients with coronary artery disease or reduced LVEF. Precautions are similar to those for flecainide (patients with renal impairment or conduction system disease, risk of proarrhythmia when increases QRS duration).

d,l-Sotalol (80–160 mg b.i.d) prevents recurrent AF as effectively as the fixed dose quinidine–verapamil combination [8], but less effectively than amiodarone. Sotalol is contraindicated in patients with significant LV hypertrophy, systolic heart failure, pre-existing QT prolongation, hypokalaemia, creatinine clearance <50 mg/mL. Drug-induced proarrhythmia with sotalol is due to excessive prolongation of the

QT interval and/or bradycardia. Careful monitoring for detection of QT prolongation and abnormal T waves is mandatory. In patients reaching a QT interval >500 ms, sotalol should be stopped or the dose reduced. The risk of proarrhythmia is increased in women, marked LV hypertrophy, severe bradycardia, ventricular arrhythmias, renal dysfunction, or electrolyte abnormalities (hypokalaemia or hypomagnesaemia).

Amiodarone (600 mg o.d. for 4 weeks, 400 mg o.d. for 4 weeks, then 200 mg o.d.) is probably the most effective drug for the prevention of recurrent AF. Amiodarone is a good therapeutic option in patients with frequent, symptomatic AF recurrences despite therapy with other antiarrhythmic drugs. Unlike most other agents, amiodarone can be safely administered in patients with structural heart disease, including patients with heart failure [9]. The risk of drug-induced torsade de pointes is lower with amiodarone than with 'pure' potassium channel blockers, possibly due to multiple ion channel inhibition. However, drug-induced proarrhythmia is seen with amiodarone, and the QT interval should be closely monitored.

Dronedarone (400 mg b.i.d.) is a multichannel blocker that inhibits the sodium, potassium, and calcium channels, and has non-competitive antiadrenergic activity. Dronedarone is less effective to maintain sinus rhythm, but also less toxic than amiodarone. In two large pivotal trials, dronedarone was superior to placebo in maintaining sinus rhythm in patients with recurrent AF [10]. The median time to the first episode of AF was 53 days in the placebo group, compared with 116 days in the dronedarone group (HR 0.75; CI 0.65–0.87; $P < 0.0001$). Dronedarone significantly reduced the ventricular rate during the first recurrence of AF or atrial flutter. In the DIONYSOS study [11] (randomized Double blind trial to evaluate efficacy and safety of drOnedarone [400 mg b.i.d.] versus amiodaroNe [600 mg q.d. for 28 days, then 200 mg q.d. thereafter] for at least 6 months for the maintenance of Sinus rhythm in patients with atrial fibrillation) including 504 patients with persistent AF, the primary composite endpoint events (recurrence of AF and study drug discontinuation) occurred in 75 % and 59 % of patients treated with dronedarone and amiodarone, respectively [hazard ratio (HR) 1.59; 95 % CI 1.28–1.98; P<0.0001]. AF recurrence was more common in the dronedarone arm compared with amiodarone (36.5 % vs. 24.3 %). Premature drug discontinuation tended to be less frequent with dronedarone (10.4 % vs. 13.3 %). The main safety endpoint occurred in 39.3 % and 44.5 % of patients treated with dronedarone and amiodarone, respectively (HR 0.80; 95 % CI 0.60–1.07; P=0.129), and was due mainly to fewer thyroid, neurological, skin, and ocular events in the dronedarone group. The safety profile of dronedarone is advantageous in patients without structural heart disease and in stable patients with heart disease. The ATHENA (A placebo-controlled, double-blind, parallel arm Trial to assess the efficacy of dronedarone 400 mg b.i.d. for the prevention of cardiovascular Hospitalisation or death from any cause in patiENts with Atrial fibrillation/atrial flutter) study [12] including 4,628 patients with paroxysmal or persistent AF or flutter and cardiovascular risk factors to be treated with dronedarone 400 mg twice daily or placebo demonstrated a reduction of cardiovascular mortality in the dronedarone group (2.7 % vs. 3.9 %; HR 0.71; 95 % CI 0.51–0.98). Post-hoc analysis also demonstrated a reduction in stroke risk in patients receiving dronedarone, which was independent of the underlying antithrombotic therapy. According to the results of the The ANtiarrhythmic trial with DROnedarone in Moderate-to-severe congestive heart failure Evaluating morbidity DecreAse (ANDROMEDA) trial dronedarone is contraindicated in NYHA class III–IV or unstable heart failure [13]. It is also contraindicated during concomitant therapy with QT-prolonging drugs, powerful CYP3A4 inhibitors, and if creatinine clearance <30 mg/mL. If used concomitantly, the dose of digitoxin/digoxin should be reduced. Elevations in serum creatinine of 0.1–0.2 mg/dL are common and do not reflect reduced renal function. Interestingly, dronedarone appears to have a low potential for proarrhythmia.

Choice of Antiarrhythmic Drugs

Antiarrhythmic therapy for recurrent AF is recommended on the basis of choosing a safer, although possibly less efficacious medication before changing to a more effective, but less safe therapy. The best options for drug therapy to suppress AF depend on the patient's comorbidities. In patients with lone AF or minimal heart disease (e.g., mild left ventricular hypertrophy), flecainide, propafenone, sotalol, and dronedarone are reasonable first-line drugs, and amiodarone and dofetilide can be considered if the first-line agents are ineffective or not tolerated. In patients with substantial left ventricular hypertrophy (left ventricular wall thickness >13 mm), the hypertrophy may heighten the risk of ventricular proarrhythmia, and the safest choice for drug therapy is amiodarone. In patients with coronary artery disease, several of the class I drugs have been found to increase the risk of death, and the safest first-line options are dofetilide, sotalol, and dronedarone, with amiodarone reserved for use as a second-line agent. In patients with heart failure, several antiarrhythmic drugs have been associated with increased mortality, and the only two drugs known to have a neutral effect on survival are amiodarone and dofetilide.

Non-antiarrhythmic Drugs

The role of non-antiarrhythmic drugs on the prevention of AF recurrences is controversial. Experimental studies indicate that angiotensin-converting enzyme (ACE) inhibitors and angiotensin receptor blockers (ARBs) have favourable effects on electrical and structural remodelling. In a meta-analysis of 11 trials that included a total of 56,308 patients, ACE inhibitors and ARBs reduced the relative risk of AF by 28 % [14]. The effect was limited to patients with left ventricular systolic dysfunction or hypertrophy. However, in a randomized clinical trial of the ARB valsartan versus placebo in 1,442 patients with structural heart disease and recurrent AF, the AF recurrence rate was approximately 50 % in both study arms, and there was no evidence that valsartan prevented

AF [15]. Therefore, whether ACE inhibitors and ARBs prevent AF is unclear, and there is insufficient evidence to support their use for the sole purpose of preventing AF. There also is some evidence that statins prevent AF, perhaps because of their anti-inflammatory effects. A systematic review of ten observational studies demonstrated a 23 % reduction in the relative risk of AF in patients treated with statins [16]. However, a meta-analysis of six randomized clinical trials concluded that statins do not prevent AF, except after open heart surgery [17]. Therefore, the available data do not support the use of statins solely for the prevention of AF. Finally, there is some evidence suggesting that aldosterone antagonists (spironolactone, eplerenone) and fish oil consumption or supplements are associated with a lower risk of the development of AF, but there is no prospective study designed to evaluate specifically this effect in patients with atrial fibrillation.

Pharmacologic Therapy for Rate Control

In patients with AF irregular rhythm and rapid ventricular rate may cause symptoms (palpitations, dyspnoea, fatigue, dizziness) and even overt heart failure (tachycardiomyopathy). Thus, the rate control therapy, prolonging the time for ventricular filling has the potential to improve haemodynamics, reducing symptoms and preventing or sometimes reversing tachycardiomyopathy. Although the optimal level of heart rate control with respect to morbidity, mortality, quality of life, and symptoms is controversial [18, 19] and remains unknown, the ESC recommend to achieve a resting heart rate between 60–80 and 90–115 bpm during moderate exercise [2].

Antiarrhythmic Drugs for Pharmacological Rate Control

Beta-blockers, non-dihydropyridine calcium channel antagonists, and digitalis are the drugs most commonly used for controlling heart rate in patients with AF (Table 5.3).

TABLE 5.3 Drugs and doses for pharmacological rate control [2]

	Intravenous administration	Usual oral maintenance dose
β-Blockers		
Metoprolol CR/XL	2.5–5 mg iv bolus over 2 min; up to 3 doses	100–200 mg o.d. (ER)
Bisoprolol	N/A	2.5–10 mg o.d
Atenolol	N/A	25–100 mg o.d
Esmolol	50–200 μg/kg/min iv	N/A
Propranolol	0.15 mg/kg iv over 1 min	10–40 mg t.i.d
Carvedilol	N/A	3.125–25 mg b.i.d.
Non-dihydropyridine calcium channel antagonists		
Verapamil	0.0375–0.15 mg/kg iv over 2 min	40 mg b.i.d. to 360 mg (ER) o.d
Diltiazem	N/A	60 mg t.i.d. to 360 mg (ER) o.d
Digitalis glycosides		
Digoxin	0.5–1 mg	0.125 mg–0.5 mg o.d
Digitoxin	0.4–0.6 mg	0.05 mg–0.1 mg o.d
Others		
Amiodarone	5 mg/kg in 1 h, and 50 mg/h maintenance	100 mg–200 mg o.d
Dronedarone[a]	N/A	400 mg b.i.d

ER extended release formulations, *N/A* not applicable
[a]Only in patients with non-permanent atrial fibrillation

Beta-adrenergic blockers are particularly useful in AF patients and ischemic heart disease. Beta-bloquers may be useful in the presence of high adrenergic tone. Dosages of the commonly used beta-blockers (bisoprolol, metoprolol, atenolol, carvedilol) are given in Table 5.3.

Non-dihydropyridine calcium channel antagonists (vera-pamil and diltiazem) are effective for acute and chronic rate control of AF. The drugs should be avoided in patients with systolic heart failure because of their negative inotropic effect.

Digoxin and digitoxin are effective for control of heart rate at rest, but not during exercise. In combination with a beta-blocker they may be effective in patients with or without heart failure. Digoxin may cause adverse effects and should there-fore be instituted cautiously. Interactions with other drugs may occur.

Amiodarone is an effective rate control drug. Nevertheless, due to the risk of severe extracardiac adverse events (e.g. pulmonary or thyroid dysfunction) amiodarone should be reserved for chronic treatment when conventional measures (beta-blockers, non-dyhydropiridine calcium channel antago-nists, digoxin) are ineffective.

Dronedarone is also effective as a rate-controlling drug for chronic treatment, but is not currently approved for permanent AF.

Other class I antiarrhythmic drugs are not effective for rate control. Sotalol should not be used solely for rate control, although its additional rate control properties may be valu-able when it is used primarily for rhythm control.

Choice of Antiarrhythmic Drugs

The choice of drugs for rate control depends on age, underly-ing heart disease, and the goal of treatment. Beta-blockers are the drugs of choice in patients with coronary artery disease and heart failure. Patients without heart disease or with hypertension can be treated with non-dihydropyridine calcium channel antagonists or beta-blockers. Verapamil, diltiazem or a beta-1 selective beta-blocker should be indicated in patients with obstructive broncho-pulmonary disease. Digoxin is fre-quently used in combination with beta-blockers or non-dihydropyridine calcium channel antagonists.

Recommendations for Long-term Rate Control

The ESC Guidelines [2] established the following recommendations for long-term rate control:

- Rate control using pharmacological agents is recommended in patients with paroxysmal, persistent, or permanent AF. The choice of medication should be individualized and the dose modulated to avoid bradycardia *(Recommendation Class I, Level B)*
- In patients who experience symptoms related to AF during activity, the adequacy of rate control should be assessed during exercise, and therapy should be adjusted to achieve a physiological chronotropic response and to avoid bradycardia. *(Recommendation Class I, Level C)*
- In pre-excitation AF, or in patients with a history of AF, preferred drugs for rate control are propafenone or amiodarone. *(Recommendation Class I, Level C)*
- It is reasonable to initiate treatment with a lenient rate control protocol aimed at a resting heart rate <110 bpm. *(Recommendation Class IIa, Level B)*
- It is reasonable to adopt a stricter rate control strategy when symptoms persist or tachycardiomyopathy occurs, despite lenient rate control: resting heart rate <80 bpm and heart rate during moderate exercise <110 bpm. After achieving the strict heart rate target, a 24 h Holter monitor is recommended to assess safety. *(Recommendation Class IIa, Level B)*
- It is reasonable to achieve rate control by administration of dronedarone in non-permanent AF except for patients with NYHA class III–IV or unstable heart failure. *(Recommendation Class IIa, Level B)*
- Digoxin is indicated in patients with heart failure and left ventricular dysfunction, and in sedentary (inactive) patients. *(Recommendation Class IIa, Level C)*
- Rate control may be achieved by administration of oral amiodarone when other measures are unsuccessful or contraindicated. *(Recommendation Class IIb, Level C)*

- Digitalis should not be used as the sole agent to control the rate of ventricular response in patients with paroxysmal AF. *(Recommendation Class III, Level B)*

References

1. Fuster V, Ryden LE, Cannom DS, et al. ACC/AHA/ESC 2006 guidelines for the management of patients with atrial fibrillation – executive summary: a report of the American College of Cardiology/ American Heart Association Task Force on Practice Guidelines and the European Society of Cardiology Committee for Practice Guidelines (Writing Committee to revise the 2001 guidelines for the management of patients with atrial fibrillation). Eur Heart J. 2006; 27:1979–2030.
2. Camm JA, Kirchhof P, Lip GYH, Schotten U, Savelieva I, Ernst S, Van Gelder IC, Al-Attar N, Hindricks G, Prendergast B, Heidbuchel H, Alfieri O, Angelini A, Atar D, Colonna P, De Caterina R, DeSutter J, Goette A, Gorenek B, Heldal M, Hohnloser SH, Kolh P, LeHeuzey JY, Ponikowski P, Rutten FR. Guidelines for the management of atrial fibrillation. Eur Heart J. 2010;31:2369–429.
3. Wyse DG, Waldo AL, DiMarco JP. A comparison of rate control and rhythm control in patients with atrial fibrillation. N Engl J Med. 2002;347:1825–32.
4. Corley SD, Epstein AE, DiMarco JP. Relationships between sinus rhythm, treatment, and survival in the Atrial Fibrillation Follow-Up Investigation of Rhythm Management (AFFIRM) study. Circulation. 2004;109:1509.
5. Tsadok MA, Jackevicius CA, Essebag V, Eisenberg MJ, Rahme E, Humphries KH, Tu JV, Behlouli H, Pilote L. Rhythm versus rate control therapy and subsequent stroke or transient ischemic attack in patients with atrial fibrillation. Circulation. 2012;126:2680–7.
6. Camm AJ, Capucci A, Hohnloser S, Torp-Pedersen C, Van Gelder IC, Mangal B, Beatch GN. A randomized active-controlled study comparing the efficacy and safety of vernakalant to amiodarone in recent onset atrial fibrillation. J Am Coll Cardiol. 2011;57:313–21.
7. Lafuente-Lafuente C, Mouly S, Longas-Tejero MA, Bergmann JF. Antiarrhythmics for maintaining sinus rhythm after cardioversion of atrial fibrillation. Cochrane Database Syst Rev. 2007;4:CD005049.
8. Fetsch T, Bauer P, Engberding R, Koch HP, Lukl J, Meinertz T, Oeff M, Seipel L, Trappe HJ, Treese N, Breithardt G. Prevention of atrial fibrillation after cardioversion: results of the PAFAC trial. Eur Heart J. 2004;25:1385–94.

9. Connolly SJ. Evidence-based analysis of amiodarone efficacy and safety. Circulation. 1999;100:2025–34.

10. Singh BN, Connolly SJ, Crijns HJ, Roy D, Kowey PR, Capucci A, Radzik D, Aliot EM, Hohnloser SH. Dronedarone for maintenance of sinus rhythm in atrial fibrillation or flutter. N Engl J Med. 2007; 357:987–99.

11. Le Heuzey JY, De Ferrari GM, Radzik D, Santini M, Zhu J, Davy JM. A short-term, randomized, double-blind, parallel-group study to evaluate the efficacy and safety of dronedarone versus amiodarone in patients with persistent atrial fibrillation: the DIONYSOS study. J Cardiovasc Electrophysiol. 2010;21:597–607.

12. Hohnloser SH, Crijns HJ, van Eickels M, Gaudin C, Page RL, Torp-Pedersen C, Connolly SJ. Effect of dronedarone on cardiovascular events in atrial fibrillation. N Engl J Med. 2009;360:668–78.

13. Kober L, Torp-Pedersen C, McMurray JJ, Gotzsche O, Levy S, Crijns H, Amlie J, Carlsen J. Increased mortality after dronedarone therapy for severe heart failure. N Engl J Med. 2008;358:2678–87.

14. Healy JS, Baranchuk A, Crystal E. Prevention of atrial fibrillation with angiotensin-converting enzyme inhibitors and angiotensin receptor blockers: a meta-analysis. J Am Coll Cardiol. 2005;45:1832.

15. Disertori M, Latini R, Barlera S. Valsartan for the prevention of recurrent atrial fibrillation. N Engl J Med. 2009;360:1606.

16. Liu T, Li L, Karantzopoulos PO. Statin use in the development of atrial fibrillation: asystematic review and meta-analysis of randomized clinical trials and observational studies. Int J Cardiol. 2008; 126:160.

17. Fauchier L, Pierre B, de Labriolle A, et al. Antiarrhythmic effect of statin therapy and atrial fibrillation a meta-analysis of randomized controlled trials. J Am Coll Cardiol. 2008;51:828.

18. AFFIRM Investigators. A comparison of rate control and rhythm control in patients with atrial fibrillation. N Engl J Med. 2002; 347:1825–33.

19. Van Gelder IC, Groenveld HF, Crijns HJ, Tuininga YS, Tijssen JG, Alings AM, Hillege HL, Bergsma-Kadijk JA, Cornel JH, Kamp O, Tukkie R, Bosker HA, Van Veldhuisen DJ, Van den Berg MP. Lenient versus strict rate control in patients with atrial fibrillation. N Engl J Med. 2010;362:1363–73.

Chapter 6
Changing the Paradigm to Understand and Manage Atrial Fibrillation

Gheorghe-Andrei Dan

Sacred Fire could not be fired with matches (Tudor Musatescu)

Abbreviations

AAD	Antiarrhythmic drug therapy
AF	Atrial fibrillation
APD	Action potential duration
CHF	Congestive heart failure
EF	Ejection fraction
HR	Heart rate
HX	History
QOL	Quality of life
RCT	Randomized controlled trials
SR	Sinus rhythm
TGFβ1	Tumor Growth Factor β1
TIA	Transient ischemic attack
WL	Wavelength

G.-A. Dan, MD, PhD, FESC, FAHA
University of Medicine "Carol Davila",
Bucharest, Romania

Internal Medicine Clinic, Cardiology Department,
Colentina University Hospital, Bucharest, Romania
e-mail: andrei.dan@gadan.ro

G.-A. Dan et al. (eds.), *Atrial Fibrillation Therapy*, Current
Cardiovascular Therapy, DOI 10.1007/978-1-4471-5475-4_6,
© Springer-Verlag London 2014

127

Rhythm Control and Rate Control Strategies in AF: A Matter of Pseudo-Equivalence

Atrial Fibrillation (AF) is an epidemic disease. In United States almost 2.5 million people suffer from AF and there is an estimate of 2.5 fold increase in the next 50 years [1]. A more recent analysis from Mayo Clinic estimates a three-fold AF upsurge in the next 50 years if a continuous increase in AF incidence is present [2]. In a contemporaneous evaluation of AF incidence and prevalence based on analysis of 8.3 million German patients, AF prevalence for 2020 is estimated at 2.661 % which represents more than twofold increase compared with previous estimates [3]. Lifetime risk for AF is high (1 in 6), even in the absence of antecedent congestive heart failure or myocardial infarction; at age 40 lifetime risk for AF reaches 25 % [4]. AF is not a benign disease: the overall mortality risk is twice that of people without AF and the arrhythmia has serious implications on the quality of life and health care costs. Certainly, the most dreaded complication of AF is the systemic thromboembolism and especially stroke. Patients with nonvalvular AF have a fivefold increase in stroke risk; this risk is up to three times in postrheumatic valvular AF. Ischemic stroke in AF is associated with an elevated mortality and morbidity; for 80 % of high risk patients the first ischemic stroke provoked by AF could be fatal or accompanied by persistent disability. Overall ischemic stroke in AF is more likely than other types of ischemic stroke to result in persistent disability or death [5] (Fig. 6.1)

Also, AF has important hemodynamic consequences due to rapid rate, irregular rhythm and abolition of atrial systole which could impede normal cardiac function with resulting clinical implications in pathological states as ischemic heart disease or heart failure.

All of the above mentioned facts argue the importance of maintaining the sinus rhythm and imply the deduction of improved outcome while maintaining sinus rhythm. Amazing, more than ten studies comparing rhythm-maintaining strategies with the more conservative rate control strategies failed to

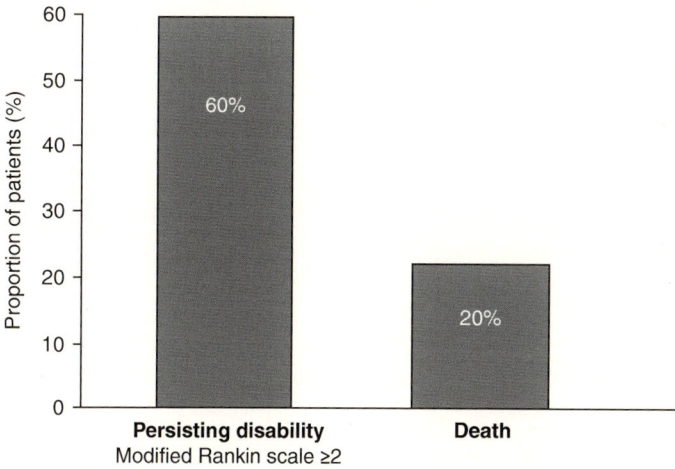

FIGURE 6.1 Outcome of first ischemic stroke in high risk patients (n: 597; high risk factors: previous stroke/TIA, age >75 years, Hx of congestive heart failure/pulmonary edema) [5]

demonstrate any long-term survival benefit. The results of the AFFIRM study [6] including 4,060 patients in two arms (rate control strategy and rhythm control strategy) refute any difference on mortality between the two strategies. Even more disturbing the AF-CHF trial [7] including 1,376 patients with AF and ejection fraction (EF) less than 35 %, a population in whom the AF deleterious effect is obvious, has shown that either sinus rhythm or rhythm control strategies are not associated with a better outcome. A meta-analysis [8] including five more important studies dealing with comparative analysis of rhythm and rate control strategies concluded that ventricular rate control combined with anticoagulant therapy is equivalent, *if not superior*, to antiarrhythmic drug therapy (AAD) to preserve sinus rhythm in patients with recurrent AF. A very recent systematic review [9] evaluated 12 randomized controlled trials (RCT) that compared pharmacological rhythm control strategy with rate-control strategy. Assuming the differences in quality and strength of evidence for these trials, the authors concluded that the two strategies are equivalent with

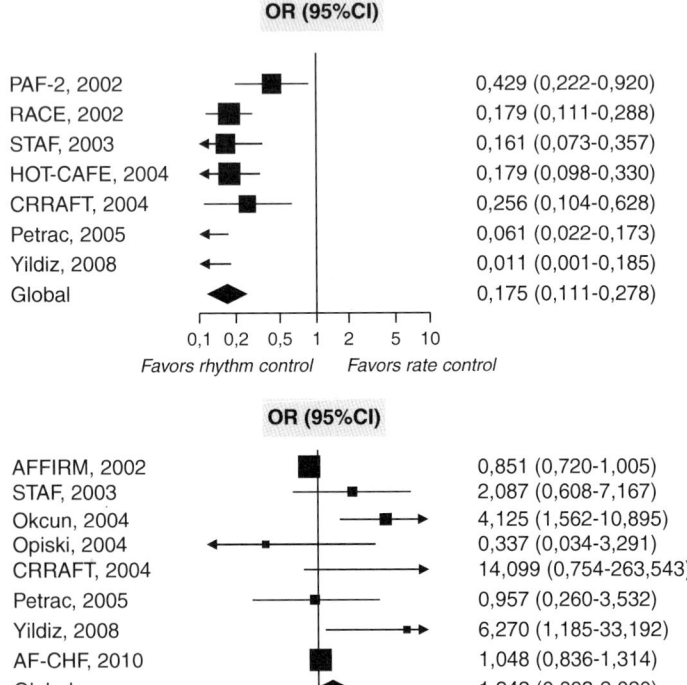

FIGURE 6.2 Maintenance of sinus rhythm (**a**) and all-cause mortality (**b**) in studies comparing rhythm and rate strategy [9]

regard to the effect on several hard outcome end-points: all-cause mortality, cardiovascular mortality and stroke. Only few studies demonstrated improvement in quality of life (QOL) or functional status with pharmacological rhythm control strategy [10, 11]. This is true despite the fact that, as expected, AAD are efficient in maintaining sinus rhythm (Fig. 6.2)

However, several studies [12–14] demonstrated with convincing evidence that rhythm control strategy is associated to reduced hospitalization (OR: 0.24, 95 % CI: 0.14–0.43). As a consequence of the *"equivalence philosophy"* both the use of AAD for maintaining sinus rhythm and the AF related hospitalizations declined [15]. Nevertheless the result of all the aforementioned trials and reviews should be interpreted very carefully in the light of the clinical practice. The real-life AF population could differ substantially from the AF – trials population; in trials the participants are younger, predominantly males and have less comorbidities. In the AFFIRM [6] trial only less than one in ten had heart failure and the mean age was below 70. Even in the AF-CHF [16] trial only one third of the participants had NYHA functional class III or IV CHF, mean age was below 68, patients had few comorbidities and only half of patients had prior hospitalizations for AF. Some interpretation bias could result from the length of the follow up. In an analysis of 26,130 patients of Quebec region from 1999 to 2007 the authors [17] observed a better long-term outcome with rhythm control strategy (HR: 0.77) versus rate control strategy. Interestingly, the curves diverged only after 5 years (which was the maximum follow-up for the AFFIRM-type studies). Another possible source of confusion could derive from the fact that both the trials and real–life patients who undergo the rhythm control strategy have the tendency to stop the anticoagulation therapy (despite the fact that in AFFIRM trial and other trials the continuation of anticoagulation was advised) with obvious implications on the outcome [18]. Use of AAD increases the possibility of silent AF; analysis of the outcome implication of silent AF made possible through recordings of implantable devices demonstrated that even short term AF episodes carry the same risk of stroke as the clinical manifest AF and that this could be one of the main causes of the *"unknown origin strokes"* which represent 25–30 % of all ischemic strokes [19]. In the last years the concept of rhythm and rate strategies equivalence was challenged by advances in ablation therapy and by improving our knowledge about arrhythmia and more subtle targets of AAD therapy. Different AF ablation procedures proved to be superior to traditional AAD in maintaining sinus rhythm and in reducing cardiovascular

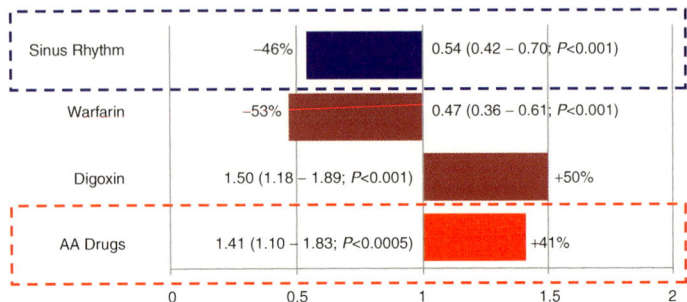

Sinus Rhythm	−46%		0.54 (0.42 – 0.70; *P*<0.001)	
Warfarin	−53%		0.47 (0.36 – 0.61; *P*<0.001)	
Digoxin	1.50 (1.18 – 1.89; *P*<0.001)		+50%	
AA Drugs	1.41 (1.10 – 1.83; *P*<0.0005)		+41%	

FIGURE 6.3 Covariates associated with survival in the AFFIRM study. Other significant factors in model: age, CAD, CHF, smoking, stroke/TIA, normal LVEF, mitral regurgitation (Modified after Corley et al. [20])

hospitalizations. Even if current studies are lacking the power to demonstrate superiority versus AAD on hard endpoints as all-cause mortality, stroke, heart failure and on long-term safety and durability, several trends in this regard were noticed. However, for a long period since now it is improbable that ablation could replace AAD in clinical practice; AF is a very prevalent disease involving one person in ten after the age of 70 and the current availability of ablation centers could not face this huge population. Moreover, phatmacological therapy is cheaper, noninvasive, nonradiant and preferred by a lot of patients. Also, the benefit and the safety of the ablation therapy in old and very old patient and in patients with important substrate modification (as in heart failure) was not yet fully established.

How to deal with the unnatural assumption of the equivalence of sinus rhythm vs. rate controlled AF? The secret is revealed by the subsequent analysis of the AFFIRM trial [20]. Looking at the covariates associated to survival it is very clear that preservation of sinus rhythm significantly decreases the risk by 46 %. This positive effect is however practically canceled by the use of the AAD which increases the risk by 41 % (Fig. 6.3).

Therefore, sinus rhythm (SR) remains the desirable target but it seems we do not dispose the appropriate tools to reach this objective. Preservation of the sinus rhythm should reduce the mortality or morbidity by halting the progression of the disease and of the consequent tendency to a permanent form of AF and dependent remodeling; also, preservation of sinus rhythm implies the decrease of the long-term embolic risk. The RECORDAF registry [21] including more than 5,000 patients demonstrated that in patients with recent onset AF who underwent rate control strategy AF progressed rapidly to permanent forms despite the fact that the outcome in these patients is driven by hospitalizations for arrhythmias or pro-arrhythmias or other cardiovascular causes and not by the AF control strategy used. Despite the fact that hypertension and heart failure are the strongest predictors for AF progression to permanent form, the rhythm control strategy is able to decrease the progression risk [22]. Why traditional AADs obscure the obvious benefit of the rhythm control strategy?

The Electrical Paradigm

Until recently AF was regarded as a pure electrical disease based on the ecg phenotype and on the main arrhythmogenesis mechanism (re-entry). Consequently, the arrhythmia was targeted with drugs illustrating the existing concept about the pure and exclusive electrical effect of the AADs. This concept is based on the somewhat simplistic approach of the so-called Singh-Vaugham-Williams classification of the AADs born in the early seventieth. There are several fatal pitfalls with the aforementioned classification and its application in clinical practice. Based on the pattern and the main mechanism for the generation of action potential the classification assumes one mechanism of action corresponding to one target/current/channel : class I blocking the sodium current (*"membrane stabilizing agents"*), class II blocking the beta adrenergic receptors, class III blocking the potassium current and consequently prolonging the action potential duration (APD) and the QT interval on ecg and class IV blocking calcium type L currents (a former class V comprising bretylium, a blocker of noradrenaline from the nerve terminals was abandoned).

Class I was further sub-divided after the drug-channel kinetics and the effect on conduction and QRS: IA for intermediate effect, IB for lack of the effect on QRS duration and the newer class IC for important effect on conduction and QRS duration. Acting on the main determinant of the conduction (sodium current and phase 0 of the APD), class I was intended mainly for lowering conduction velocity while class III AAD, with minimal effects on conduction, was intended mainly for lowering excitability. As always with forcing things in standard boxes, i.e. drug classes, the individual components of the different AAD classes not only share actions very different from the class they belong to, but also common actions with other classes. For instance, Quinidine, a class IA drug exhibits, in fact, potassium channel blocking effects at lower dosage and sodium blocker properties at higher dosages. Propafenone and Sotalol both share beta-blocker (class II) actions and Amiodarone, constrained to class III, has class I, class II and class IV actions together with other important actions (as the interference with thyroid hormones). The multiple electrophysiological actions of one drug could interfere with the main class action to modify the anti-arrhythmic efficacy or the safety of the individual compound, as assumed from the class effect. Amiodarone is by far the most effective anti-arrhythmic drug and it is very likely that this virtue is linked to the multiple targets of actions; Dronedarone, a similar compound lacking the iodine moiety is less effective than amiodarone in preventing AF recurrences [23]. Another element, with important clinical implications, obscured in the simplicity of the Singh-Vaugham-Williams classification is related to the channel kinetics of the drug. Some drugs (quinidine, Sotalol) manifest *"reverse use dependence"* which means that the predominant effect is observed at lower rates, while others (lidocaine, flecainide, propafenone) manifest *"use dependence"* which means that the electrophysiological effect is predominant at higher rates. The former is responsible for QT prolongation and *torsade des pointes* during bradycardia and the second is responsible for anti-tachycardia efficiency. The subtle electrophysiological, pharmacokinetic and pharmacodynamic properties of AADs have more than a simple academic meaning. Without this detailed knowledge, nor the efficacy neither the safety are warranted. Table 6.1 presents the main mechanism, pharmacological properties and clinical effects of the classical AADs intended for rhythm control strategy.

However, despite the extensive pharmacological knowledge, applying to individual patient with AF the general principles of the electrical paradigm, based exclusively on the genesis of the APD and the Singh-Vaugham-Williams classification, represents an empirical strategy with a high rate of clinical failure. For example it seems very attractive to treat AF with drugs decreasing conduction (class IC), but in clinical practice amiodarone (class III, acting on excitability) proved to have more consistent effects on maintaining SR; yet, even with amiodarone the benefit is moderate (65 % of patients without documented recurrences at less than 2 years [25], a percent of benefit further diminished by the number of patients keeping spontaneously the SR during the same follow-up). Last but not the least, several substances (digoxin, adenosine, magnesium sulphate…) with known antiarrhythmic effects are not and could not be listed with the too sketchy Singh-Vaugham-Williams classification. Efforts were made in the last decade of the past century to diminish the empiricism of the antiarrhythmic therapy and to anticipate the efficacy and undesirable effects of the existing AAD. The most remarkable result in this direction is the "Sicilian Gambit" classification [26] (the name was given after the Taormina (Sicily) meeting of the authorities in the field of arrhythmias). In fact the "Sicilian Gambit" is more a thinking algorhythm modality than a classification (this is the meaning of the term "gambit" with the analogy to chess). The *Sicilian Gambit* was not very popular among clinicians mainly because it is quite complicated and descriptive and implies the knowledge of arrhythmias mechanisms, pharmacology of the AAD and ECG; however, the *Sicilian Gambit* represents not only the most valuable tool to treat efficiently and safely an individual patient with AADs but also it proved to be the

TABLE 6.1 Antiarrhythmic drugs used to convert AF and to maintain sinus rhythm (Modified after Zimetbaum [24])

Antiarrhythmic drug	Channel current or receptor	Pharmacokinetics, metabolism, dosage	Adverse effects (cardiac and noncardiac)	Selected drug interactions
Quinidine, 1918	I_{Na}, I_{Kr}, I_{to}, I_{Ach}, α	Hepatic CYP3A4 (70 %), renal (30 %); dose: sulfate, 600 mg three times a day; gluconate, 324–648 mg every 8 h; reduced dose for renal failure	Thrombocytopenia, cinchonism, pruritus, rash QRS prolongation with toxic doses, torsades de pointes (not dose related)	↑ digoxin and amiodarone concentrations; quinidine inhibits CYP2D6 and may ↑ drugs metabolized by this enzyme (e.g., ↑ effect of tricyclic antidepressants, haloperidol, some β-blockers, fluoxetine, narcotics); quinidine metabolism is inhibited by cimetidine; quinidine metabolism is ↑ by phenobarbital, phenytoin, and rifampicin
Disopyramide, 1962	I_{Na}, I_{Kr}, acetylcholine	Renal/hepatic CYP3A4; dose: 100–400 mg every 8–12 h; maximum dose, 800 mg/24 h; reduced dose for renal or hepatic dysfunction	Anticholinergic (contraindicated for narrow-angle glaucoma): dry mouth, urinary retention, constipation, blurry vision Congestive heart failure exacerbation, torsades de pointes	None

Propafenone, 1976	I_{Na}, β	Hepatic: 150–300 mg every 8 h or sustained release 225–425 mg twice a day	Metallic taste, dizziness Atrial flutter with 1:1 conduction; VT; may unmask Brugada-type ST elevation; contraindicated with coronary disease	May ↓ the metabolism of warfarin; ↑ digoxin levels
Flecainide, 1975	I_{Na}	Renal/hepatic CYP2D6; 50–100 mg twice a day, maximum dose 300–400 mg/day	Dizziness, headache, visual blurring Atrial flutter with 1:1 conduction; VT; may unmask Brugada-type ST elevation; contraindicated with coronary disease	May ↑ digoxin levels; flecainide levels are ↑ by amiodarone, haloperidol, quinidine, cimetidine, and fluoxetine
Sotalol, 1992, 2000 (AF)	I_{Kr}, β	Renal: 80–120 mg twice a day; maximum dose 240 mg twice a day	Bronchospasm Bradycardia, torsades de pointes	No significant interactions

(continued)

TABLE 6.1 (continued)

Antiarrhythmic drug	Channel current or receptor	Pharmacokinetics, metabolism, dosage	Adverse effects (cardiac and noncardiac)	Selected drug interactions
Dofetilide, 2000 (US only)	I_{Kr}	Renal/hepatic CYP3A4; CrCL >60 ml/min (500 μg twice a day), CrCl 40–60 ml/min (250 μg twice a day), CrCl 20–39 ml/min (125 μg twice a day)	Torsades de pointes	Contraindicated with verapamil, ketoconazole, cimetidine, megestrol, prochlorperazine, and trimethoprim; hydrochlorothiazide ↑ dofetilide levels; must discontinue amiodarone at least 3 month before dofetilide initiation
Ibutilide (i.v.), 1995	I_{Kr}, I_{Na} agonist	Hepatic CYP3A4; 1 mg intravenous over 10 min; repeat after 10 min, if necessary	Nausea Torsades de pointes	None

| Amiodarone, 1967 | I_{Kr}, I_{Na}, I_{Ca}, β, α, acetylcholine | Hepatic; half-life 50 days: oral load 10 g over 7–10 days, then 400 mg for 3 weeks, then 200 mg/day for AF; maintenance dose of 400 mg/day for VT; dose: reduced load if bradycardia or QT prolongation; intravenous: 150–300 mg bolus, then 1 mg/min infusion for 6 h followed by 0.5 mg/min thereafter | Pulmonary (acute hypersensitivity pneumonitis, chronic interstitial infiltrates); hepatitis; thyroid (hypo- or hyperthyroidism); photosensitivity; blue-gray skin discoloration with chronic high dose; nausea; ataxia; tremor; alopecia Sinus bradicardia | Inhibits CYP450 enzymes; ↑ concentrations of warfarin, digoxin, cyclosporine, alprazolam, carbamazepine, statins (simvastatin), phenytoin, and quinidine; ↑ the effect of dabigatran, but does not appear to be clinically relevant |

(continued)

TABLE 6.1 (continued)

Antiarrhythmic drug	Channel current or receptor	Pharmacokinetics, metabolism, dosage	Adverse effects (cardiac and noncardiac)	Selected drug interactions
Dronedarone, 2009	I_{Kr}, I_{Na}, I_{Ca}, β, α, acetylcholine	Renal, hepatic, gastrointestinal; 400 mg twice a day	Anorexia; nausea; hepatotoxicity Bradycardia	Inhibits CYP3A4; ↑ levels of alprazolam, carbamazepine, dihydropyridine, cyclosporine, statins, digoxin; verapamil (but not diltiazem) ↑ dronedarone levels; contraindicated in the presence of strong CYP3A4 inhibitors such as ketoconazole, itraconazole, cyclosporine, clarithromycin, and ritonavir; ↑ effects of dabigatran

| Vernakalant (i.v.), 2010 (Europe only) | I_{Kur}, I_{Na} | Dysgeusia; sneezing; paresthesia | Hypotension (contraindicated in presence of severe aortic stenosis, class 3 or 4 congestive heart failure, or preexisting hypotension); QT prolongation; increased risk of ventricular arrhythmias in patients with congestive heart failure |

basis for changing the paradigm of the antiarrhythmic therapy. The *Sicilian Gambit* assumes that there are specific arrhythmogenic mechanisms at the cell level and at the heart level: enhanced and abnormal automatism, triggered activity (early after depolarization and delayed after depolarization), re-entry and others, less important. These mechanisms are responsible for the specific type of arrhythmias as characterized clinically and on ecg. It is also assumed that alteration of one or few electrophysiological properties will be sufficient to terminate the arrhythmia and to prevent further recurrences; among these properties one is more susceptible to therapeutic intervention and with fewest undesirable effects. This one is called *the vulnerable parameter.* For each vulnerable parameter there are one or more components most likely to modulate the mechanism (channels, pumps, carriers, receptors, regulators…). The most appropriate cellular or molecular target for drug action represents the *critical component.* Besides these important considerations regarding efficiency when using AADs, several important safety issues should be considered: effects on cardiac contractility, on sinus rhythm and extracardiac effects of the drug together with the effects on the surface ecg (as a marker of action or toxicity). The concepts of "vulnerable parameter" and "critical components" remain a cornerstone when looking for better understanding of arrhythmogenesis and for new AAD with improved efficiency and safety.

Unfortunately, even with more profound knowledge of the general arrhythmias electrical mechanisms and pharmacology of current AADs, applying the "electrical paradigm" – i.e. focusing only on the electrical mechanism of the arrhythmia and of AADs action – will preserve the empiricism of the rhythm control strategy in AF and the therapeutic approach with current membrane acting agents will be limited by adverse effects and low efficacy. Safety remains the main concern with classical/old AADs. This became very clear after publication of the Cardiac Arrhythmia Suppression Trial (CAST) results. In this trial [27], including 3,549 patients, aimed to prove a decrease in sudden cardiac death mortality in post-myocardial infarction patients with ventricular ectopy, prematurely closed because of safety reasons, the "new" potent class IC AADs encainide and flecainide increased the cardiovascular mortality with a relative risk of 2.5, despite the fact that a huge percent of treated patients remained free of arrhythmias [28]. There were two important lessons from CAST study. First is that treating surrogate end-points empirically could have disastrous effect. Second, as said once Philippe Coumel, "*(classical/old) AADs are poisons doing occasionally well*". A recent Cochrane systematic review [29] evaluating AAD for maintaining sinus rhythm, which includes 20,771 patients from 56 studies, demonstrates increase in mortality with class IA AAD (OR: 2.39) and with Sotalol (OR: 2.47) despite reduction in AF recurrences (which is also true for beta blockers). All AADs showed increased withdrawal because of adverse effects and with the exception of amiodarone, Dronedarone and Propafenone all increased significantly the risk of proarrhythmia. When compared with class I AAD, amiodarone showed a nonsignificant trend to lower mortality and a significant reduction of recurrences rate (OR: 0.36). The authors failed to demonstrate any benefit on clinically relevant outcomes (heart failure or systemic embolism).

Because of the serious adverse effects encountered with AAD and not only because of the advances in interventional antiarrhythmic therapy, the pharmacological treatment of arrhythmias and especially of AF became less attractive in clinical practice [17]. The public impact was huge as Druin Burch noted in 2010 in "*New Scientist*" that "*AAD cost more American lives than the Vietnam War*" [30]. Also, in the AF management guidelines, with the exception of amiodarone (and to a lesser extent Sotalol and Dronedarone), the AADs are recommended for patients with normal heart or minimally structural diseased heart [31].

It appears that a changing in paradigm is necessary: moving from adapting the disease to the existing drugs toward adapting drugs to intimate subtle and individual mechanisms of the disease.

Atrial Fibrillation as a Multifactorial Syndrome: The Holistic Approach

The AF electrocardiographic pattern is only the final pheno-type of a multifactorial complex syndrome resulting in mul-tiple diverse pathways. This complexity implies that it is more important to manage the patient with AF than managing AF itself, as it was seen the classical historical approach.

Causality Network of AF: Risk Factors for Initiation and Perpetuation, Markers, Modulators and Factors of Progression

There were described many risk factors associated to AF; some of them proved to have a causal relationship with AF. Identifying them and interfering with them, the prevention or halting the progression of AF is possible. There are also risk markers associated with development of AF. They indicate the processes and the persons prone to the development of AF and are, therefore, valuable in its primary or secondary prevention. Table 6.2 presents the most important risk factors and markers for AF subject to intervention for the preven-tion of AF [32]; however, substantial evidence from random-ized trials regarding the possible benefit is still missing and the design of such trials is difficult to conceive.

Atrial fibrillation pathophysiology could be regarded as a two-step process. In the first part different known and unknown risk factors act individually or together, through separate or shared mechanisms, to modify the cardiac sub-strate morphologic, functional and electrical properties. Some of the risk factors or mechanisms are signaled by specific markers. There are several fewer common physiological mechanisms which could initiate or perpetuate AF (fibrosis, inflammation, channel remodeling...). The remodeling pro-cess is also influenced by modulating factors [33] (such as age, genetic predisposition, autonomic nervous system function,

TABLE 6.2 Risk factors and markers for atrial fibrillation

Validated risk factors	Less validated risk factors	New risk factors	AF markers
Age	Obesity/BMI	Birth weight	PR interval
Male gender	Pulse pressure	Preclinical atherosclerosis	Murmur
Concomitant conditions	Height	Psychological determinant	Hemodynamic stress
• Hypertension	Sleep apnea syndrome		• BNP, ANP
• Valve disease	Subclinical hyperthyroidism		Inflammation
• Heart failure	Alcohol consumption		• CRP
• Coronary artery disease	Chronic kidney disease		• Il6
• Myocardial infarction	Excessive endurance sports		• TNF-α
• Diabetes	COPD		Cardiac damage
Associated risk factors	Coffee		Troponins
• Family history			
• AF susceptible loci (GWAS)			

GWAS genome wide associated studies; *COPD* chronic obstructive pulmonary disease (Modified after Kirchhof et al. [32])

hormonal and metabolic factors). Once initiated by this common pathway, AF perpetuates itself, remodeling the substrate; in this way not only the AF has the tendency to be transformed in more permanent forms, but also AF becomes itself a factor and marker of risk for the initiating processes with consequent outcome implications (Fig. 6.4).

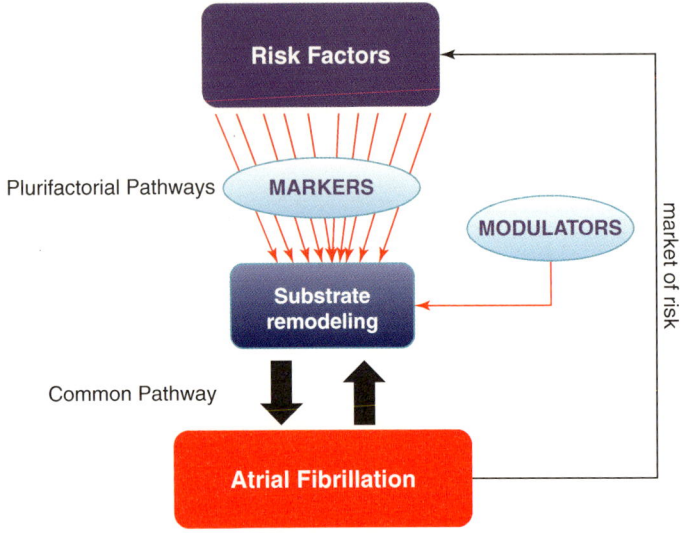

FIGURE 6.4 Causal relationships of AF showing the plurifactorial pathways and the common pathway of initiation and perpetuation

Therefore, AF is a progressive disease with the tendency to end up in a permanent form and delaying to control the process from the very beginning could explain the failure of latter attempts to control the rhythm and recurrences [34]. In the Canadian Registry of Atrial Fibrillation which included 757 patients at the first documented AF episode, the rate of progression to chronic AF was 8 % in the first year and increased slowly, but continuously to 24.7 % at 5 years [35]. As a proof of AF self-perpetuation capacity, from 71 patients with lone paroxysmal or persistent AF of the Olmsted County population (Minnesota), during a follow-up period of 30 years, 22 progressed to permanent AF [36]. However, it seems that remodeling and progression are not compulsory for all AF patients. In a study including 330 patients with documented paroxysmal AF and implanted for bradyar-rhythmias with pacemakers having the possibility to record AF burden, only 24 % progressed to persistent AF during a follow-up period less than 1 year; this progression was highly correlated with the presence of structural heart disease. In the remaining patients without associated cardiac disease there was no increase in AF burden despite a higher density of triggers (atrial premature beats) and a higher likelihood of daily AF episodes [37]. The EuroHeartSurvey investigators [38] identified five important predictors for AF progression grouped under the "*HATCH score*" (hypertension, age above 75, transient ischemic attack (TIA) or stroke, chronic obstructive pulmonary disease and heart failure, each characteristic receiving one point, with the exception of TIA/stroke and heart failure receiving two points). Nearly a half of patients progress to persistent AF when HATCH score is ≥5 compared to only 6 % when HATCH score is 0. Because AF is a frequent condition, it becomes important to select those at higher risk to develop it as they represent excellent candidates for prophylactic measures. Several clinical based models have been developed aiming to elaborate scores with a better prediction value and to indicate how to incorporate new biomarkers for the further improvement of the prediction[39–42]. Recently, a simplified score [43] was validated (C-index 0.718) based exclusively on few clinical characteristics (age, weight, height, systolic blood pressure, alcohol use, and smoking) readily to be applied in people without heart disease in whom ecg or echographic evaluation are not always available; analysis was based on predictors from Women's Health Study. These scores are working well, but the sensibility is quite limited indicating a true higher risk mainly to those who subsequently will demonstrate an AF burden of 60–80 % [44]. The AF risk is modulated by an important heritable component. This is not surprising as the cardiac electrophysiology is governed by channels function and by the genes that encode channels; alterations in atrial channels function (loss- or gain-of-function) modify the atrial APD characteristics and could increase AF susceptibility [45]. There is a long research history in the field of genetic basis of AF beginning with the discovery in 1943 of a rare form of autosomal-dominant genetic form of atrial fibrillation in three brothers

(Wolf cited by [46]). Some rare variants with Mendelian inheritance have strong effect but confer low population – attributable risk while others, with a complex inheritance pattern, are common and, despite a weak effect, confer a high population-attributable risk. Between the two extremes there is a continuous spectrum of combinations of common and rare variants with a large aggregate effect [46]. With improvement in genetic technology and decreasing in cost, more than ten genes or family of genes associated with increased risk of AF were discovered and after identification of the first three common susceptibility loci on chromosomes 4, 16 and 1, six new different common susceptibility loci were discovered using genome-wide association studies (GWAS) [47]. When genes involved in the control of cardiac expressed channels are involved, loss or gain in channel function could increase the susceptibility for AF through several mechanisms: shortening of the atrial refractory period, increased atrial APD and susceptibility for triggered activity, abnormal and heterogeneous cell to cell impulse propagation (disturbances of connexin and gap-junction function). GWAS made possible to identify several genetic mechanisms that implicate genes without previously known role in AF pathophysiology as those controlling transcription factors involved in cardiopulmonary development and signaling molecules or modulating atrial fibrosis [47]. Finally, some genetic polymorphism could interfere indirectly with AF through modulation of drug effect. For example the β1 adrenoreceptor genotype Arg389Arg is associated with increased heart rate during AF and increased cardioversion potency of flecainide [48], while angiotensin converting enzyme DD or ID genotypes are highly predictive for failure of AADs [49, 46]. The genetic heritage combines different genetic variants with other risk factors to generate different degrees of AF susceptibility (the so called "*two-hit hypothesis*" [46]).

There is only a modest improvement of the AF prediction calculated with traditional clinical score scales through adding a genetic risk score based on known susceptibility alleles [50, 43]. However, improving genetic methodology the discovery

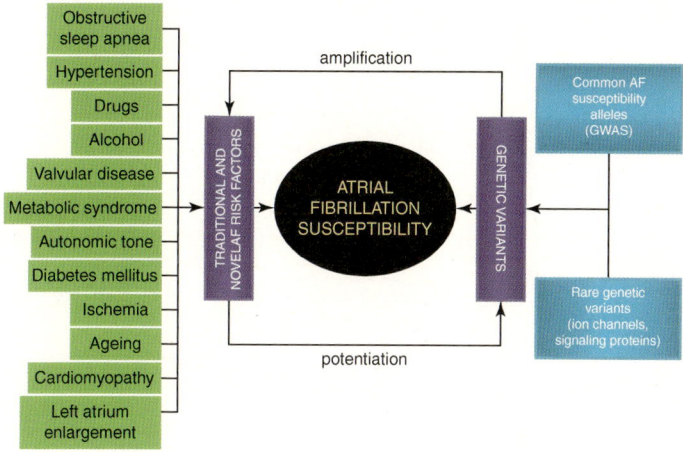

FIGURE 6.5   The two-hit hypothesis: combined effect of traditional risk factors and genetic factors in AF pathogenesis. Genetic variants could amplify the pathogenic effect of traditional risk factors and on their turn, risk factors could unmask or increase the phenotypic action of the genetic variants (Modified after Darbar and Roden [46])

of new variants with large effect or revealing new intergenic or environment-genic interactions will probably modify this contribution [44] (Fig. 6.5).

The Common Pathway of AF Initiation and Perpetuation: The Electrophysiological Mechanism

To be produced AF needs a suitable modified substrate and a shutter (trigger) unmasking the electrical inhomogeneity of the modified atrial substrate and initiating the reentry which is the main engine of AF. The proportional contribution of the substrate and of the trigger to the initiation and particularly the perpetuation of AF varies between individual types of AF and for the same patient varies during the time course of the disease. More the contribution of the substrate, higher the progression to permanent forms of AF. The reverse is true for rare occasions in which AF is dependent almost exclusively

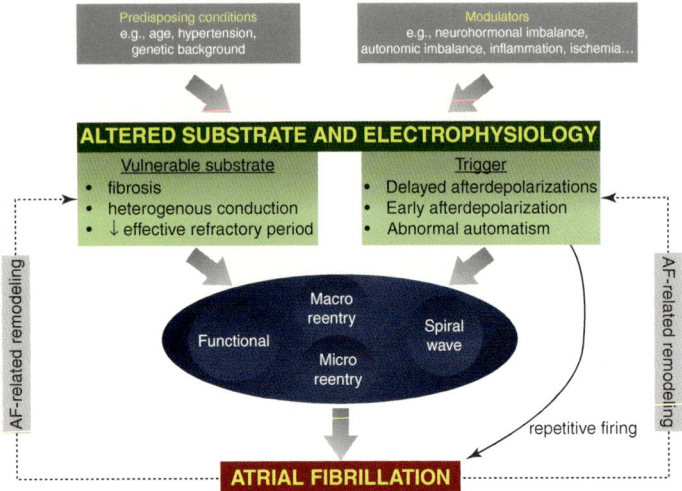

FIGURE 6.6 The "common pathway" of AF initiation and perpetuation [52] and [53]

on triggers from automatic foci inside pulmonary veins [51] and is usually a paroxysmal form. An already modified atrial substrate, but yet unsuitable to initiate reentry, could be acutely "activated" by modulators as neuroumoral imbalance, autonomic nervous system imbalance, ischemia or inflammation. Reentry in AF is of functional "*leading* circle" type (i.e. not around a fixed anatomic substrate) or spiral wave type. An initial unstable macro-reentrant circuit is transformed through electrical remodeling (decrease in effective refractoriness and in conduction velocity) in more stable microcircuits; the presence of multiple microcircuits with small wavelength on a limited area makes AF more stable and difficult to terminate (Fig. 6.6).

Several subtle mechanisms initiated by AF itself compete for creating the prerequisites of AF perpetuation – *Atrial fibrillation begets atrial fibrillation(Wijffels 1995)*. Increase in HR after AF initiation increases sarcoplasmic calcium concentration. As an adaptive reaction to limit calcium cytotoxic effect, the calcium current I_{CaL} is inactivated rapidly. This effect turns in a maladaptive reaction as all APD, wavelength (WL) and rate adaptation of the atrial APD are decreased as a consequence. If the increased HR persists, the initial more reversible decrease in I_{CaL} becomes more profound through transcriptional and translational interventions, downregulating calcium-channel protein units [52]. Despite the fact that alterations in calcium current are an essential component of the electrical remodeling, I_{CaL} is not downregulated in some forms of AF (as in ventricular dysfunction [54]) and it is not the sole electrophysiological component of atrial remodeling. Increase in inward rectifier current I_{K1} makes the resting atrial membrane potential more negative, increasing the sodium current availability and stabilizing the reentry [53]. Increase in I_{KAch}, a current mediating the vagal effects, further decreases APD. I_{KATP}, a current sensitive to ATP, seems to play a role in the atrial electrical remodeling of the ischemia associated AF. There is a complex picture of the atrial currents and channels remodeling in AF which makes difficult the interpretation of the physiologic role. Some potassium currents (as the ultra-rapid atria-specific potassium current I_{Kur}) are not upregulated, but downregulated in AF as a contra regulatory reaction to prevent excessive shortening in refractoriness. Not only the sarcolemmal channels are remodeled in AF, but, also, the contact between cells is modified. There are functional and structural alterations of the junction-gaps which support AF perpetuation through decreased conduction velocity and increased dispersion of APD. The connexin 43 (most abundant component of the gap-junction channel), 40 and 45 are downregulated and, also, there is a lateral redistribution of these components from the normal head-to-head with obvious increase in anisotropic conduction.

Electrical remodeling involves, also, intracellular channels and signaling proteins. There are important alterations of calcium sarcoplasmic reticulum handling in AF. In AF a calcium leak from the sarcoplasmic reticulum was observed [55] and this promotes the substrate for triggered activity (delayed after depolarization) which could initiate or maintain AF. Calcium

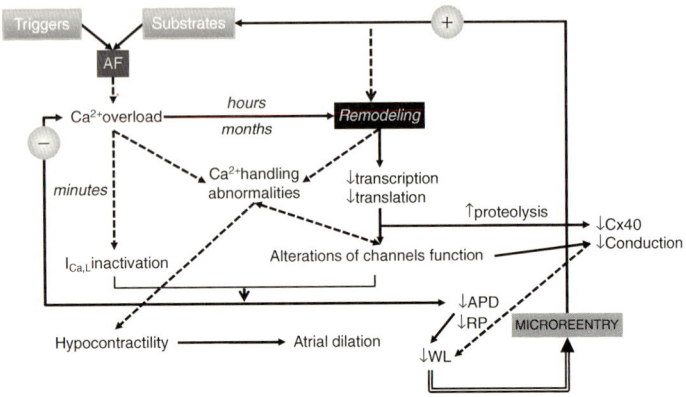

FIGURE 6.7 Atrial electro-remodeling and perpetuation of AF (Modified after Nattel et al. [52])

leak is determined by phosphorylation of sarcoplasmic reticulum ryanodine receptor RyR2 due to activation of Calcium/Calmodulin dependent/protein-kinase II (CaMKII) [56]. Atrial myocite seems to be more sensitive to small amounts of calcium leak because of an increased diastolic voltage-calcium coupling gain [55]. Micro RNA, small noncoding molecules which negatively modify the function of target mRNA, were demonstrated recently to play a role in potassium channel and calcium handling remodeling [53] (Fig. 6.7).

The Common Pathway of AF Initiation and Perpetuation: Fibrosis and Inflammation

Fibrosis is very common in AF and was documented in all types of AF including "lone atrial fibrillation". There is a two-way relationship between AF and fibrosis, although to determine the pathogenic importance of fibrosis to AF initiation and perpetuation is still challenging [57]. Fibrosis could be the result of the insult of the underlying heart disease or of the age itself as there is a 6 % risk per year of developing myocardial fibrosis after the age of 65 (Shenassa M., 2011, personal communication). On the other hand there is now increasing evidence that AF could be itself the arrhythmic manifestation of a group of diseases called *"fibrotic atrial cardiomyopathy (FACM)"* [58] which has several expressions of the fibrotic burden and clinical manifestations (ranging from asymptomatic to multiple arrhythmic presentations). There is a correlation between extracellular cardiac matrix composition and quantity and AF persistence [57]. Atrial fibrosis is proarrhythmogenic through several mechanisms linked to the structural and electrophysiological inhomogeneity and to the fibroblast-myocite coupling: decrease in conduction velocity and promoting reentry (i.e. maintaining rotors), triggered activity initiation and triggered activity propagation [59, 60]. Additionally, fibroblast mechanical stretch modulates the myocite electrical activity (*mechanoelectrical feedback*) [61]. Atrial fibrosis could be promoted in the absence of a detectable underlying structural disease through several known mechanisms (including genetic predisposition, atrial structural remodeling/dilatation, inflammation) and probably more unknown mechanisms. Evidences derived from direct histologic examination or imaging using delayed-enhancement MRI showed that in lone AF there is a substrate characterized by increased collagen synthesis and mild to moderate fibrosis [62]. There are several promoters of atrial fibrosis, many of them intervening in progression of other cardiovascular diseases. Renin-angiotensin-aldosterone system plays a central role in profibrotic processes and transforming growth factor β1 (TGFβ1), is a powerful signaling molecule of the profibrotic cascade, and a key factor for atrial fibrosis; overexpression of TGFβ1 causes selective atrial fibrosis, functional heterogeneity and AF propensity [57]. Fibroblasts and myocite interact during the remodeling process and Angiotensin II and TGFβ1 amplify each other's generation. During mechanical stretch angiotensin II, angiotensin II receptors A1 and TGFβ1are overexpressed and, as a result, additional profibrotic molecules are produced [57]. This molecular autocrine and paracrine cross-talk governing atrial remodeling secondary to atrial dilatation or to increase in intraatrial pressure

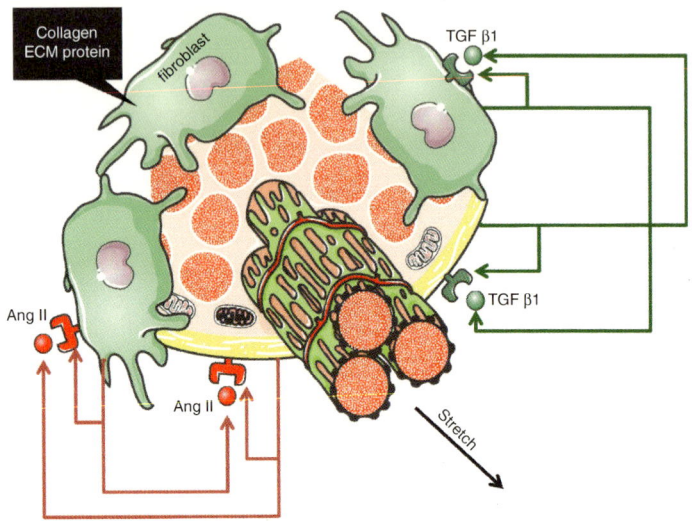

Figure 6.8 Interrelations between cardiomyocyte and fibroblast mediated by the crosstalk between angiotensin II and TGFβ1. *ECM* extracellular matrix

seems to be very sensitive to the model of atrial deformation resulting in different forms of fibrotic pattern [63] (Fig. 6.8)

Abnormal calcium signaling plays a role in TGFβ1 production and fibrotic remodeling. An increased calcium influx mediated through fibroblast transient receptor potential (TRP) channel was observed in AF patients and contributes to TGFβ1 mediated fibrosis [53]. Micro RNA involved in electrical remodeling controls, also, some TRP expression creating thus a link between the structural and electrical remodeling.

Inflammation seems also to take part in the AF generation and perpetuation. Atrial biopsies revealed inflammation in patients with AF and the condition is associated with increased level of some inflammatory markers [64]. High sensitive-C reactive protein, TNFα, interleukin 6, VCAM1,

ICAM 1, monocyte chemo-attraction molecule 1 were found elevated in patients with AF and some of them predict new-onset AF. Also, markers of the oxidative stress are increased in patients with AF. Again, angiotensin II has a central role in modulating the inflammatory process in AF. Despite a definite role in AF cardiac remodeling, normalization of inflammatory markers after arrhythmia ablation suggests inflammation as an effect and mechanism for perpetuation, but not as cause [65].

The Present and Future of the Antiarrhythmic Therapy

Preservation of the sinus rhythm is an essential long-term objective in atrial fibrillation to reduce mortality, stroke incidence, morbidity and total AF burden and to improve the quality of life. To address this objective the modern antiarrhythmic therapy should take into consideration the complex pathophysiology of AF and the individual mechanisms for the initiation and the perpetuation of AF in a particular patient. Treating the electrocardiogram is no longer acceptable. With current limitations of the old and classical AAD, the indications for rhythm control strategy are somewhat subjective and difficult to implement. This explains the decline in the AADs prescription observed after publication of the AFFIRM trial [17]. The most accepted indications for rhythm control strategy with current AAD are younger age, symptomatic episodes, active patient, recent onset paroxysmal AF, minimal underlying cardiac disease, curable cause and minimal atrial remodeling [66]. This perspective will change with newer, better targeted therapy, focusing on the "vulnerable" parameters of AF initiation and perpetuation. This modern therapy in accord with the transformation of our understanding paradigm of atrial fibrillation should fill the gap of the last three decades (Table 6.3).

TABLE 6.3 Present and future rhythm therapy of AF (Modified after Heijman et al. [53])

Target	Present	Future	Comment
Replication of amiodarone efficacy	Amiodarone	Celivarone	Dronedarone contraindicated in heart failure and permanent AF
	Dronedarone	Budiodarone	Celivarone Phase IIb of clinical study
Excitability, conduction, ectopic activity	Class IC AADs	Atrial selective I_{Na} inhibition	
	Vernakalant	Ca^{+2} handling normalization	
	Ranolazine		
Refractoriness, reentry	Class III AADs (dofetilide, sotalol, amiodarone, dronedarone)	Atrial selective ion-channel modulation	NTC-801 (I_{Kach}) XEN-D0103 (I_{Kur})
Remodeling, fibrosis, inflammation	ACEi, ARBs, Statin	Ca^{+2} signaling (calpain, calcineurin)	Pirfenidone was approved in pulmonary idiopathic fibrosis
	Beta-blockers	Kinases and phosphatases	
	Spironolactone	Pirfenidone	
	PUFA (?)	MicroRNA modulation	

Calcium handling	Carvedilol	Carvedilol analogues (VK-II86, CS-I-34, CS-I-59)	Carvedilol reduces SR calcium leak through antioxidant properties and inhibitory RyR2 actions
		JTV-519 and its derivative S107	JTV-519: benzothiazepine derivative; stabilizes RyR2 complex
		Dantrolene	Dantrolene: stabilizes RyR2
		SEA 0400	SEA0400: Inhibition of NCX (Na-Ca exchanger)
Gap junction	Rotigaptide (discontinued)	Danegaptide	Normalizes connexin expression
		Adenoviral mediated gene therapy with Cx 40 or Cx 43	Decreases fibrosis
Mechano-electric coupling	–	GsMTx-4 (Gadolinium, Streptomycin)	Acts on stretch activated channels

ACEi angiotensin converting enzyme inhibitors, *ARB* angiotensin receptor blocker, *Cx* connexin, *PUFA* poly-unsaturated fatty acids

References

1. Go AS, Hylek EM, Phillips KA, Chang Y, Henault LE, Selby JV, Singer DE. Prevalence of diagnosed atrial fibrillation in adults: national implications for rhythm management and stroke prevention: the AnTicoagulation and Risk Factors in Atrial Fibrillation (ATRIA) study. JAMA. 2001;285(18):2370–5.

2. De S, Go AS, Hylek EM, Phillips KA, Chang Y, Henault LE, Selby JV. Secular trends in incidence of atrial fibrillation in Olmsted County, Minnesota, 1980 to 2000, and implications on the projections for future prevalence. Circulation. 2006;114:119–25.

3. Wilke T, Groth A, Mueller S, Pfannkuche M, Verheyen F, Linder R, Maywald U, Bauersachs R, Breithardt G. Incidence and prevalence of atrial fibrillation: an analysis based on 8.3 million patients. Europace. 2013;15(4):486–93.

4. Lloyd-Jones DM, Wang TJ, Leip EP, Larson MG, Levy D, Vasan RS, D'Agostino RB, Massaro JM, Beiser A, Wolf PA, Benjamin EJ. Lifetime risk for development of atrial fibrillation: the Framingham heart study. Circulation. 2004;110(9):1042–6.

5. Gladstone DJ, Bui E, Fang J, Laupacis A, Lindsay MP, Tu JV, Silver FL, Kapral MK. Potentially preventable strokes in high-risk patients with atrial fibrillation who are not adequately anticoagulated. Stroke. 2009;40(1):235–40.

6. Wyse DG, Waldo AL, DiMarco JP, Domanski MJ, Rosenberg Y, Schron EB, Kellen JC, Greene HL, Mickel MC, Dalquist JE, Corley SD. A comparison of rate control and rhythm control in patients with atrial fibrillation. New Engl J Med. 2002;347(23):1825–33.

7. Talajic M, Khairy P, Levesque S, Connolly SJ, Dorian P, Dubuc M, Guerra PG, Hohnloser SH, Lee KL, Macle L, Nattel S, Pedersen OD, Stevenson LW, Thibault B, Waldo AL, Wyse DG, Roy D. Maintenance of sinus rhythm and survival in patients with heart failure and atrial fibrillation. J Am Coll Cardiol. 2010;55(17):1796–802.

8. de Denus S, Sanoski CA, Carlsson J, Opolski G, Spinler SA. Rate vs rhythm control in patients with atrial fibrillation: a meta-analysis. Arch Intern Med. 2005;165(3):258–62.

9. Al-khatib SM, Lapointe NA, Chatterjee R. Treatment of atrial fibrillation. Eff Health Care Program. 2013; Comparativ(119).

10. Vora A, Karnad D, Goyal V, Naik A, Gupta A, Lokhandwala Y, Kulkarni H, Singh BN. Control of heart rate versus rhythm in rheumatic atrial fibrillation: a randomized study. J Cardiovas Pharmacol Ther. 2004;9(2):65–73.

11. Opolski G, Torbicki A, Kosior DA, Szulc M, Wozakowska-Kaplon B, Kolodziej P, Achremczyk P. Rate control vs rhythm control in patients with nonvalvular persistent atrial fibrillation: the results of the polish how to treat chronic atrial fibrillation (HOT CAFE) study. Chest. 2004;126(2):476–86.

12. Carlsson J, Miketic S, Windeler J, Cuneo A, Haun S, Micus S, Walter S, Tebbe U. Randomized trial of rate-control versus rhythm-control in persistent atrial fibrillation: the Strategies of Treatment of Atrial Fibrillation (STAF) study. J Am Coll Cardiol. 2003;41(10):1690–6.

13. Brignole M, Menozzi C, Gasparini M, Bongiorni MG, Botto GL, Ometto R, Alboni P, Bruna C, Vincenti A, Verlato R. An evaluation of the strategy of maintenance of sinus rhythm by antiarrhythmic drug therapy after ablation and pacing therapy in patients with paroxysmal atrial fibrillation. Eur Heart J. 2002;23(11):892–900.

14. Petrac D, Radić B, Radeljić V, Hamel D, Filipović J. Ventricular pacing vs dual chamber pacing in patients with persistent atrial fibrillation after atrioventricular node ablation: open randomized study. Croat Med J. 2005;46(6):922–8.

15. Martin-Doyle W, Essebag V, Zimetbaum P, Reynolds MR. Trends in US hospitalization rates and rhythm control therapies following publication of the AFFIRM and RACE trials. J Cardiovasc Electrophysiol. 2011;22(5):548–53.

16. Roy D, Talajic M, Nattel S, Wyse DG, Dorian P, Lee KL, Bourassa MG, Arnold JMO, Buxton AE, Camm AJ, Connolly SJ, Dubuc M, Ducharme A, Guerra PG, Hohnloser SH, Lambert J, Le Heuzey J-Y, O'Hara G, Pedersen OD, Rouleau J-L, Singh BN, Stevenson LW, Stevenson WG, Thibault B, Waldo AL. Rhythm control versus rate control for atrial fibrillation and heart failure. New Engl J Med. 2008;358(25):2667–77.

17. Ionescu-Ittu R, Abrahamowicz M, Jackevicius CA, Essebag V, Eisenberg MJ, Wynant W, Richard H, Pilote L. Comparative effectiveness of rhythm control vs rate control drug treatment effect on mortality in patients with atrial fibrillation. Arch Int Med. 2012;172(13):997–1004.

18. Zimetbaum P. Is rate control or rhythm control preferable in patients with atrial fibrillation? An argument for maintenance of sinus rhythm in patients with atrial fibrillation. Circulation. 2005;111(23):3150–6. discussion 3156–7.

19. Healey JS, Connolly SJ, Gold MR, Israel CW, Van Gelder IC, Capucci A, Lau CP, Fain E, Yang S, Bailleul C, Morillo CA, Carlson M, Themeles E, Kaufman ES, Hohnloser SH. Subclinical atrial fibrillation and the risk of stroke. New Engl J Med. 2012;366(2):120–9.

20. Corley SD, Epstein AE, DiMarco JP, Domanski MJ, Geller N, Greene HL, Josephson RA, Kellen JC, Klein RC, Krahn AD, Mickel M, Mitchell LB, Nelson JD, Rosenberg Y, Schron E, Shemanski L, Waldo AL, Wyse DG. Relationships between sinus rhythm, treatment, and survival in the Atrial Fibrillation Follow-Up Investigation of Rhythm Management (AFFIRM) study. Circulation. 2004;109(12):1509–13.

21. Camm AJ, Breithardt G, Crijns H, Dorian P, Kowey P, Le Heuzey J-Y, Merioua I, Pedrazzini L, Prystowsky EN, Schwartz PJ, Torp-Pedersen C, Weintraub W. Real-life observations of clinical outcomes

with rhythm- and rate-control therapies for atrial fibrillation RECORDAF (Registry on Cardiac Rhythm Disorders Assessing the Control of Atrial Fibrillation). J Am Coll Cardiol. 2011;58(5):493–501.

22. De Vos CB, Breithardt G, Camm AJ, Dorian P, Kowey PR, Le Heuzey J-Y, Naditch-Brûlé L, Prystowsky EN, Schwartz PJ, Torp-Pedersen C, Weintraub WS, Crijns HJ. Progression of atrial fibrillation in the REgistry on Cardiac rhythm disORDers assessing the control of atrial fibrillation cohort: clinical correlates and the effect of rhythm-control therapy. Am Heart J. 2012;163(5):887–93.

23. Le Heuzey J-Y, De Ferrari GM, Radzik D, Santini M, Zhu J, Davy J-M. A short-term, randomized, double-blind, parallel-group study to evaluate the efficacy and safety of dronedarone versus amiodarone in patients with persistent atrial fibrillation: the DIONYSOS study. J Cardiovasc Electrophysiol. 2010;21(6):597–605.

24. Zimetbaum P. Antiarrhythmic drug therapy for atrial fibrillation. Circulation. 2012;125(2):381–9.

25. Roy D, Talajic M, Dorian P, Connolly S, Eisenberg MJ, Green M, Kus T, Lambert J, Dubuc M, Gagné P, Nattel S, Thibault B. Amiodarone to prevent recurrence of atrial fibrillation. Canadian trial of atrial fibrillation investigators. New Engl J Med. 2000;342(13):913–20.

26. The 'Sicilian Gambit'. A new approach to the classification of antiarrhythmic drugs based on their actions on arrhythmogenic mechanisms. The task force of the working group on arrhythmias of the European Society of Cardiology. Eur Heart J. 1991;12(10):1112–31.

27. Echt DS, Liebson PR, Mitchell LB, Peters RW, Obias-Manno D, Barker AH, Arensberg D, Baker A, Friedman L, Greene HL. Mortality and morbidity in patients receiving encainide, flecainide, or placebo. The cardiac arrhythmia suppression trial. New Engl J Med. 1991;324(12):781–8.

28. Epstein AE, Hallstrom AP, Rogers WJ, Liebson PR, Seals AA, Anderson JL, Cohen JD, Capone RJ, Wyse DG. Mortality following ventricular arrhythmia suppression by encainide, flecainide, and moricizine after myocardial infarction. The original design concept of the Cardiac Arrhythmia Suppression Trial (CAST). JAMA. 1993; 270(20):2451–5.

29. Lafuente-Lafuente C, Longas-Tejero MA, Bergmann J-F, Belmin J. Antiarrhythmics for maintaining sinus rhythm after cardioversion of atrial fibrillation. Cochrane Database Syst Rev. 2012;5:CD005049.

30. Burch D. Do not harm. New Sci. 2010;Juin 12, no. Opinion 969.

31. Camm AJ, Lip GYH, De Caterina R, Savelieva I, Atar D, Hohnloser SH, Hindricks G, Kirchhof P, Bax JJ, Baumgartner H, Ceconi C, Dean V, Deaton C, Fagard R, Funck-Brentano C, Hasdai D, Hoes A, Knuuti J, Kolh P, McDonagh T, Moulin C, Popescu BA, Reiner Z, Sechtem U, Sirnes PA, Tendera M, Torbicki A, Vahanian A, Windecker S, Vardas P, Al-Attar N, Alfieri O, Angelini A, Blömstrom-

Lundqvist C, Colonna P, De Sutter J, Ernst S, Goette A, Gorenek B, Hatala R, Heidbüchel H, Heldal M, Kristensen SD, Le Heuzey J-Y, Mavrakis H, Mont L, Filardi PP, Ponikowski P, Prendergast B, Rutten FH, Schotten U, Van Gelder IC, Verheugt FWA. 2012 focused update of the ESC Guidelines for the management of atrial fibrillation: an update of the 2010 ESC Guidelines for the management of atrial fibrillation. Developed with the special contribution of the European heart rhythm association. Eur Heart J. 2012; 33(21):2719–47.

32. Kirchhof P, Lip GYH, Van Gelder IC, Bax J, Hylek E, Kaab S, Schotten U, Wegscheider K, Boriani G, Brandes A, Ezekowitz M, Diener H, Haegeli L, Heidbuchel H, Lane D, Mont L, Willems S, Dorian P, Aunes-Jansson M, Blomstrom-Lundqvist C, Borentain M, Breitenstein S, Brueckmann M, Cater N, Clemens A, Dobrev D, Dubner S, Edvardsson NG, Friberg L, Goette A, Gulizia M, Hatala R, Horwood J, Szumowski L, Kappenberger L, Kautzner J, Leute A, Lobban T, Meyer R, Millerhagen J, Morgan J, Muenzel F, Nabauer M, Baertels C, Oeff M, Paar D, Polifka J, Ravens U, Rosin L, Stegink W, Steinbeck G, Vardas P, Vincent A, Walter M, Breithardt G, Camm AJ. Comprehensive risk reduction in patients with atrial fibrillation: emerging diagnostic and therapeutic options–a report from the 3rd atrial fibrillation competence NETwork/European heart rhythm association consensus conference. Europace. 2012;14(1):8–27.

33. Wyse DG, Gersh BJ. Atrial fibrillation: a perspective: thinking inside and outside the box. Circulation. 2004;109(25):3089–95.

34. Cosio FG, Aliot E, Botto GL, Heidbüchel H, Geller CJ, Kirchhof P, De Haro J-C, Frank R, Villacastin JP, Vijgen J, Crijns H. Delayed rhythm control of atrial fibrillation may be a cause of failure to prevent recurrences: reasons for change to active antiarrhythmic treatment at the time of the first detected episode. Europace. 2008; 10(1):21–7.

35. Kerr CR, Humphries KH, Talajic M, Klein GJ, Connolly SJ, Green M, Boone J, Sheldon R, Dorian P, Newman D. Progression to chronic atrial fibrillation after the initial diagnosis of paroxysmal atrial fibrillation: results from the Canadian registry of atrial fibrillation. Am Heart J. 2005;149(3):489–96.

36. Jahangir A, Lee V, Friedman PA, Trusty JM, Hodge DO, Kopecky SL, Packer DL, Hammill SC, Shen W-K, Gersh BJ. Long-term progression and outcomes with aging in patients with lone atrial fibrillation: a 30-year follow-up study. Circulation. 2007;115(24):3050–6.

37. Saksena S, Hettrick DA, Koehler JL, Grammatico A, Padeletti L. Progression of paroxysmal atrial fibrillation to persistent atrial fibrillation in patients with bradyarrhythmias. Am Heart J. 2007; 154(5):884–92.

38. de Vos CB, Pisters R, Nieuwlaat R, Prins MH, Tieleman RG, Coelen R-JS, van den Heijkant AC, Allessie MA, Crijns HJGM. Progression

from paroxysmal to persistent atrial fibrillation clinical correlates and prognosis. J Am Coll Cardiol. 2010;55(8):725–31.

39. Benjamin EJ, Levy D, Vaziri SM, D'Agostino RB, Belanger AJ, Wolf PA. Independent risk factors for atrial fibrillation in a population-based cohort. The Framingham heart study. JAMA. 1994;271(11):840–4.

40. Psaty BM, Manolio TA, Kuller LH, Kronmal RA, Cushman M, Fried LP, White R, Furberg CD, Rautaharju PM. Incidence of and risk factors for atrial fibrillation in older adults. Circulation. 1997;96(7):2455–61.

41. Schnabel RB, Sullivan LM, Levy D, Pencina MJ, Massaro JM, D'Agostino RB, Newton-Cheh C, Yamamoto JF, Magnani JW, Tadros TM, Kannel WB, Wang TJ, Ellinor PT, Wolf PA, Vasan RS, Benjamin EJ. Development of a risk score for atrial fibrillation (Framingham Heart Study): a community-based cohort study. Lancet. 2009;373(9665):739–45.

42. Chamberlain AM, Agarwal SK, Folsom AR, Soliman EZ, Chambless LE, Crow R, Ambrose M, Alonso A. A clinical risk score for atrial fibrillation in a biracial prospective cohort (from the Atherosclerosis Risk in Communities [ARIC] study). Am J Cardiol. 2011;107(1):85–91.

43. Everett BM, Cook NR, Conen D, Chasman DI, Ridker PM, Albert CM. Novel genetic markers improve measures of atrial fibrillation risk prediction. Eur Heart J. 2013;34(29):2243–51.

44. Lubitz SA, Husser D. Genomic risk scores in atrial fibrillation: predicting the unpredictable? Eur Heart J. 2013;34(29):2227–9.

45. Darbar D. Genetics of atrial fibrillation: rare mutations, common polymorphisms, and clinical relevance. Heart Rhythm. 2008;5(3):483–6. the official journal of the Heart Rhythm Society.

46. Darbar D, Roden DM. Genetic mechanisms of atrial fibrillation: impact on response to treatment. Nat Rev Cardiol. 2013;10(6):317–29.

47. Ellinor PT, Lunetta KL, Albert CM, Glazer NL, Ritchie MD, Smith AV, Arking DE, Müller-Nurasyid M, Krijthe BP, Lubitz SA, Bis JC, Chung MK, Dörr M, Ozaki K, Roberts JD, Smith JG, Pfeufer A, Sinner MF, Lohman K, Ding J, Smith NL, Smith JD, Rienstra M, Rice KM, Van Wagoner DR, Magnani JW, Wakili R, Clauss S, Rotter JI, Steinbeck G, Launer LJ, Davies RW, Borkovich M, Harris TB, Lin H, Völker U, Völzke H, Milan DJ, Hofman A, Boerwinkle E, Chen LY, Soliman EZ, Voight BF, Li G, Chakravarti A, Kubo M, Tedrow UB, Rose LM, Ridker PM, Conen D, Tsunoda T, Furukawa T, Sotoodehnia N, Xu S, Kamatani N, Levy D, Nakamura Y, Parvez B, Mahida S, Furie KL, Rosand J, Muhammad R, Psaty BM, Meitinger T, Perz S, Wichmann H-E, Witteman JCM, Kao WHL, Kathiresan S, Roden DM, Uitterlinden AG, Rivadeneira F, McKnight B, Sjögren M, Newman AB, Liu Y, Gollob MH, Melander O, Tanaka T, Stricker BHC, Felix SB, Alonso A, Darbar D, Barnard J, Chasman DI, Heckbert SR, Benjamin EJ, Gudnason V, Kääb S. Meta-analysis identifies six new susceptibility loci for atrial fibrillation. Nat Genet. 2012;44(6):670–5.

48. Nia AM, Caglayan E, Gassanov N, Zimmermann T, Aslan O, Hellmich M, Duru F, Erdmann E, Rosenkranz S, Er F. Beta1-adrenoceptor polymorphism predicts flecainide action in patients with atrial fibrillation. PloS One. 2010;5(7):e11421.

49. Darbar D, Motsinger AA, Ritchie MD, Gainer JV, Roden DM. Polymorphism modulates symptomatic response to antiarrhythmic drug therapy in patients with lone atrial fibrillation. Heart Rhythm. 2007;4(6):743–9.

50. Lubitz SA, Yin X, Fontes JD, Magnani JW, Rienstra M, Pai M, Villalon ML, Vasan RS, Pencina MJ, Levy D, Larson MG, Ellinor PT, Benjamin EJ. Association between familial atrial fibrillation and risk of new-onset atrial fibrillation. JAMA. 2010;304(20):2263–9.

51. Haïssaguerre M, Jaïs P, Shah DC, Takahashi A, Hocini M, Quiniou G, Garrigue S, Le Mouroux A, Le Métayer P, Clémenty J. Spontaneous initiation of atrial fibrillation by ectopic beats originating in the pulmonary veins. New Engl J Med. 1998;339(10):659–66.

52. Nattel S, Burstein B, Dobrev D. Atrial remodeling and atrial fibrillation: mechanisms and implications. Circ Arrhythm Electrophysiol. 2008;1(1):62–73.

53. Heijman J, Voigt N, Dobrev D. New directions in antiarrhythmic drug therapy for atrial fibrillation. Future Cardiol. 2013;9(1):71–88.

54. Workman AJ, Pau D, Redpath CJ, Marshall GE, Russell JA, Norrie J, Kane KA, Rankin AC. Atrial cellular electrophysiological changes in patients with ventricular dysfunction may predispose to AF. Heart Rhythm. 2009;6(4):445–51.

55. Voigt N, Li N, Wang Q, Wang W, Trafford AW, Abu-Taha I, Sun Q, Wieland T, Ravens U, Nattel S, Wehrens XHT, Dobrev D. Enhanced sarcoplasmic reticulum Ca2+ leak and increased Na+-Ca2+ exchanger function underlie delayed afterdepolarizations in patients with chronic atrial fibrillation. Circulation. 2012;125(17):2059–70.

56. Neef S, Dybkova N, Sossalla S, Ort KR, Fluschnik N, Neumann K, Seipelt R, Schöndube FA, Hasenfuss G, Maier LS. CaMKII-dependent diastolic SR Ca2+ leak and elevated diastolic Ca2+ levels in right atrial myocardium of patients with atrial fibrillation. Circ Res. 2010;106(6):1134–44.

57. Burstein B, Nattel S. Atrial fibrosis: mechanisms and clinical relevance in atrial fibrillation. J Am Coll Cardiol. 2008;51(8):802–9.

58. Kottkamp H. Fibrotic atrial cardiomyopathy: a specific disease/syndrome supplying substrates for atrial fibrillation, atrial tachycardia, sinus node disease, AV node disease, and thromboembolic complications. J Cardiovasc Electrophysiol. 2012;23(7):797–9.

59. Miragoli M, Salvarani N, Rohr S. Myofibroblasts induce ectopic activity in cardiac tissue. Circ Res. 2007;101(8):755–8.

60. Morita N, Sovari AA, Xie Y, Fishbein MC, Mandel WJ, Garfinkel A, Lin S-F, Chen P-S, Xie L-H, Chen F, Qu Z, Weiss JN, Karagueuzian HS. Increased susceptibility of aged hearts to ventricular fibrillation

during oxidative stress. Am J Physiol Heart Circ Physiol. 2009;297(5):H1594–605.

61. Kamkin A, Kiseleva I, Lozinsky I, Scholz H. Electrical interaction of mechanosensitive fibroblasts and myocytes in the heart. Basic Res Cardiol. 2005;100(4):337–45.

62. Kottkamp H. Human atrial fibrillation substrate: towards a specific fibrotic atrial cardiomyopathy. Eur Heart J. 2013;Facm I.

63. MacKenna D, Summerour SR, Villarreal FJ. Role of mechanical factors in modulating cardiac fibroblast function and extracellular matrix synthesis. Cardiovasc Res. 2000;46(2):257–63.

64. Marcus GM, Smith LM, Ordovas K, Scheinman MM, Kim AM, Badhwar N, Lee RJ, Tseng ZH, Lee BK, Olgin JE. Intracardiac and extracardiac markers of inflammation during atrial fibrillation. Heart Rhythm. 2010;7(2):149–54.

65. Marcus GM, Smith LM, Glidden DV, Wilson E, McCabe JM, Whiteman D, Tseng ZH, Badhwar N, Lee BK, Lee RJ, Scheinman MM, Olgin JE. Markers of inflammation before and after curative ablation of atrial flutter. Heart Rhythm. 2008;5(2):215–21. the official journal of the Heart Rhythm Society.

66. Camm AJ, Camm CF, Savelieva I. Medical treatment of atrial fibrillation. J Cardiovasc Med (Hagerstown, Md). 2012;13(2):97–107.

Chapter 7
Guidelines and Current Recommendations in Atrial Fibrillation

Antoni Martínez-Rubio and Gheorghe-Andrei Dan

Introduction

Atrial fibrillation (AF) is a very common arrhythmia characterized by chaotic electrical atrium activation reflected in the electrocardiogram by variable R-R intervals and absence of P waves.

Different researches have demonstrated and increasing prevalence related to age and also to various comorbidities (e.g. arterial hypertension). Since this arrhythmia diminishes quality of life and severely increases stroke and mortality risk, it is a major challenge for any society with major individual, social and economic impact. Therefore, several guidelines for its management have been proposed by the major cardiologic societies.

A. Martínez-Rubio, MD, PhD, MsHM, FESC, FACC (✉)
Department of Cardiology, University Hospital of Sabadell,
Parc Taulí s/n, E-08208 Sabadell, Barcelona, Spain
e-mail: 22917amr@comb.cat

G.-A. Dan, MD, PhD, FESC, FAHA
Internal Medicine Clinic and Department of Cardiology,
Colentina University Hospital, Bucharest, Romania

Department of Internal Medicine and Cardiology,
Faculty of Medicine, University of Medicine and
Pharmacy Carol Davila, Bucharest, Romania

G.-A. Dan et al. (eds.), *Atrial Fibrillation Therapy*, Current
Cardiovascular Therapy, DOI 10.1007/978-1-4471-5475-4_7,
© Springer-Verlag London 2014

This chapter summarizes the key points proposed by the European Society of Cardiology (ESC) in its last update of AF-guidelines [1] which are more extensive and separately commented in other chapters of this book.

New Recommendations

For the Diagnosis of AF

Opportunistic screening for AF in patients ≥65 years using pulse-taking followed by an ECG is advised for diagnosing the arrhythmia previous to the occurrence of its complications in those individuals with an irregular pulse (class I B recommendation).

For the Definition of Valvular AF

ESC guidelines consider that AF related to rheumatic valvular disease (mainly mitral stenosis) or prosthetic heart valves should be described as "valvular AF". Thus, the term "non-valvular AF" includes the other AF causes. However, the definition does not precisely describe the level of valvular affection considered imperatively necessary for "valvular AF" definition. Usually, physicians understand, thus, the term "valvular AF" for clinically significant valvular affection.

For Stroke Risk Assessment

In contrast to focus on identifying "high-risk" patients, and since anticoagulation and antiplatelet therapy increase the risk of bleeding, the most recent ESC guideline focus on identification of "truly-low-risk" patients with AF who do not need any antithrombotic therapy.

Because the CHADS$_2$ (**C**ongestive heart failure, **H**ypertension, **A**ge ≥75, **D**iabetes mellitus and **S**troke

CHAD$_2$DS$_2$-VASC
Assessment of Thromboembolic Risk

Variable	Points
Congestive heart failure / LV dysfunction	1
Hypertension	1
Age >75	2
Diabetes mellitus	1
Stroke/TIA/TE	2
Vascular disease (Prior MI, AoD, PAD)	1
Age 65-74	1
Sex category (female)	1

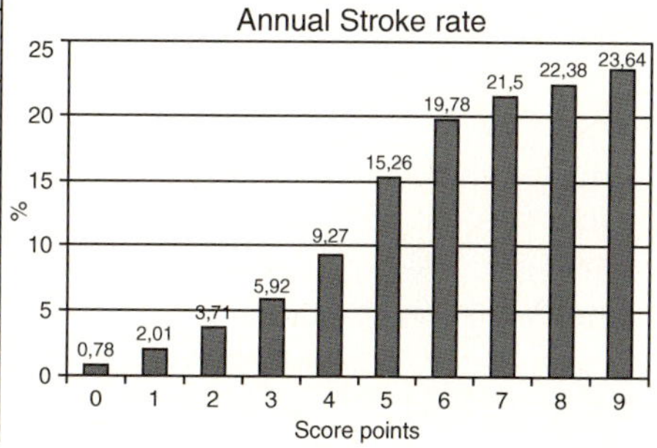

Annual Stroke rate — bar chart of % versus Score points (0–9): 0,78; 2,01; 3,71; 5,92; 9,27; 15,26; 19,78; 21,5; 22,38; 23,64

FIGURE 7.1 Validation of the assessment of stroke risk using CHA$_2$DS$_2$-VASc score in a cohort of 73,538 patients (Modified from reference [3]). Abbreviations: *AoD* Aortic plaques, *LV* left ventricular, *MI* myocardial infarction, *PAD* peripheral artery disease, *TIA* transient ischemic attack, *TE* previous thromboembolism

(doubled)) score has limitations and it does not considers well-known independent risk factors for stroke (e.g. vascular disease), the ESC suggests to use a new stroke risk assessment method with the CHA$_2$DS$_2$-VASc (**C**ongestive heart failure/left ventricular dysfunction, **H**ypertension, **A**ge >75 (doubled), **D**iabetes mellitus, **S**troke (doubled), **V**ascular disease, **A**ge 65–74 and **S**ex category (female)) score, which has been validated in a diverse cohorts of patients [2, 3] (Fig. 7.1). Importantly, the term congestive heart failure refers to patients with documented moderate-to-sever systolic dysfunction or patients with recent decompensated heart failure requiring hospitalization (irrespective of ejection fraction). Female gender is an independent stroke risk factor unless in persons of age <65 years with lone AF.

In contrast to older, conflicting data, thyroid disease (or hyperthyroidism) is not considered to be an independent stroke risk factor.

For Stroke Risk Prevention in Non-valvular AF

Obviously the best prevention of the stroke risk is to eliminate the arrhythmia and to maintain the sinus rhythm. However, since this can only be achieved in an small portion of patients and it cannot be precisely predicted who and when will have a recurrence, the broad majority of patients will need chronic anticoagulation in the course of their life. However, since truly low-risk patients exist (i.e. age <65 and lone AF (including female)), the new guideline only recommends effective stroke prevention therapy with adjusted-dose VKA (INR of 2–3) or with one of the new oral anticoagulation drugs (NOACs (dabigatran, rivaroxaban, apixaban)) for those persons who present a CHA_2DS_2-VASc score ≥ 2 (class I, level A). If the score is 0, no antithrombotic therapy and either no antiplatelet therapy is recommended (Fig. 7.2) since these patients have a very low stroke-risk, which is counterbalanced by bleeding risk with the mentioned drugs (class I, level B). Importantly, the rate of major bleeding and of intracranial hemorrhage is similar for aspirin and warfarin although the antiplatelet drug is significantly less effective than the antithrombotic drug for stroke prevention [4]. For those patients who present a CHA_2DS_2-VASc score of 1, oral anticoagulation (with VKA or NOACs) should be considered, based upon an assessment of the risk of bleeding complications and patient preferences (class IIa, level A).

NOACs should be considered rather than adjusted-dose of VKA for most patients with non-valvular AF, based on their net clinical benefit (class IIa, Level A). In addition, NOACs should be used if difficulties in keeping INR in therapeutic range exist, as well as in patients who experience side effects o VKAs or have inability to attend or undertake INR monitoring (class I, level B).

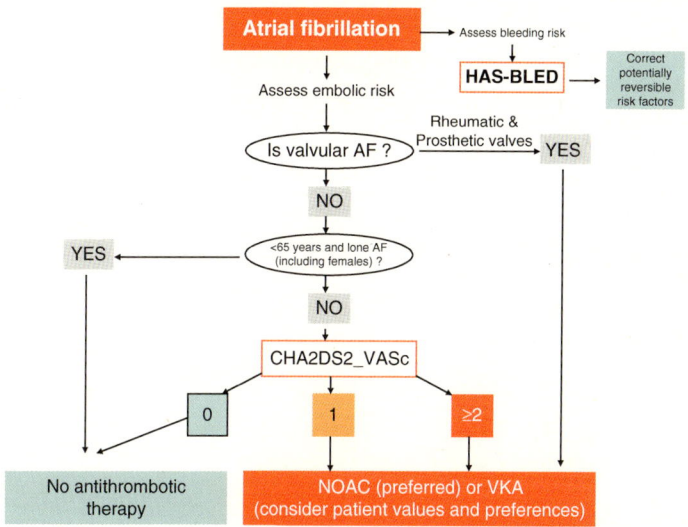

FIGURE 7.2 Choice of anticoagulant in atrial fibrillation based in reference [1]. Abbreviations: *AF* atrial fibrillation, *CHA₂DS₂-VASc* see text, *HAS-BLED* see text, *NOAC* novel oral anticoagulants, *VKA* vitamin K antagonists

Those patients who refuse the use of any OAC may be treated using combination therapy with aspirin 75–100 mg/day plus clopidogrel 75 mg/day (where there is a low risk of bleeding) or less effectively with aspirin alone (class IIa, level B).

For pericardioversion prevention of thromboembolism of those patients with AF ≥48 h of duration, or when the duration of AF is unknown, VKA treatment or dabigatran is recommended for ≥3 weeks prior to and for ≥4 weeks after cardioversion, regardless of the method (electrical or pharmacological) (class I, level B). Irrespective of the apparent maintenance of sinus rhythm following cardioversion, those patients with risk factors for stroke or AF recurrence should be lifelong treated with oral anticoagulation drugs (class I, level B).

TABLE 7.1 Assessment of bleeding risk [HAS-BLED] in atrial fibrillation patients recommended by ESC [1]

HAS-BLED	Score
Hypertension (systolic blood pressure > 160 mmHg)	1
Abnormal renal and liver function (one point each)	1 or 2
Stroke	1
Bleeding tendency/predisposition	1
Labile INRs (if on warfarin)	1
Elderly (e.g. age > 65)	1
Drugs (e.g. NSAIDs, aspirin) or alcohol abuse (one point for each category)	1 or 2
Maximum score	9

For Bleeding Risk Assessment

In addition to stroke risk also bleeding risk assessment is mandatory. To simplify the last, the European Society of Cardiology (since 2010 ESC guidelines on AF), the Canadian Cardiovascular Society and the consensus document on bleeding in AF, prepared by the European Heart Rhythm Association (EHRA) and the ESC Working Group on Thrombosis recommend to use the HAS-BLED score rather than other less practical or more complicated scores (Table 7.1). The HAS-BLED score has been validated in different cohorts of patients, correlates well with the risk of intracranial bleeding and should be used for risk assessment of all patients with AF [4]. A score which is ≥3 suggests the need of caution, regular review of bleeding risk and efforts to correct potentially reversible factors, but not to exclude patients from anticoagulation therapy.

New Recommendations for Anticoagulant Drugs

Vitamin K antagonists (VKA) are useful but have several clinical limitations, which have been detailed by Martínez-Rubio et al. in another chapter of this book. The new ESC guidelines suggest that the use of the NOACs should be preferred for the broad majority of patients with AF because these agents are "at least" non-inferior to warfarin, with a better safety profile than VKA (especially the three drugs have consistently shown a reduction of intracranial bleedings). However, since there is still limited experience, a strict adherence to only approved indications and post-marketing surveillance are mandatory. In, addition, concerns in some populations (e.g. very elderly patients, multiple comorbidities, polypharmacy, etc.), compliance issues, lack of specific antidotes and lack of broad clinical experience (e.g. perioperative management), and of the immediate cost of the drug still exist. However, diverse cost-efficacy studies (inclusive from official agencies) are being reported in different countries and present results favoring the use of these drugs based on a long-term perspective.

Actually, two types of NOAC have been presented: oral direct thrombin inhibitors (e.g. dabigatran) and oral direct factor Xa inhibitors (e.g. rivaroxaban, apixaban, edoxaban, etc.). Thus, the NOAC block only one single step of the coagulation cascade (in contrast to multiple vitamin-K dependent coagulation factors which are affected by use of VKA).

The available data of randomized phase III trials comparing the use of warfarin versus dabigatran (RE-LY) [5], ribaroxaban (ROCKET-AF) [6] and APIXABAN (ARISTOTLE) [7] are summarized in Tables 7.2 and 7.3. Importantly, patients with severe renal impairment (creatinine clearance <30 mL/min) have been excluded from all these clinical trials and ESC guidelines do not recommend the use of the NOACs in this population. Up to now, only indirect comparisons of these drugs are possible. Recently, a practical and extensive guide on the use of the NOACs in patients with non-valvular atrial fibrillation has been published [8].

Stroke Prevention in Patients Undergoing Catheter Ablation

Ablation during uninterrupted NOAC carries a small theoretical risk if a bleeding occurs. However, interruption of oral anticoagulation or switching to other therapies

TABLE 7.2 Key differences in design and patient characteristics between the three available randomized phase III trials comparing warfarin versus dabigatran (RE-LY) [5], rivaroxaban (ROCKET-AF) [6] and apixaban (ARISTOTLE) [7] in patients with non-valvular atrial fibrillation. Abbreviations: *AF* atrial fibrillation, *ASA* aspirin, *CHADS2* see text, *CHF* congestive heart failure, *TIA* transitoric ischemic attack, *SE* systemic thromboembolism, *VKA* vitamin-K antagonist

Key Differences

	RELY	ROCKET AF	ARISTOTLE
Design	PROBE	BLINDED	BLINDED
Randomized	18,113	14,264	18,201
Mean Age (yrs)	71	73	70
Male (%)	64	61	65
CHADS 2 Score (mean)	2.1	3.5	2.1
0–1 (%)	32	0	34
2 (%)	35	14	35.8
3 + (%)	33	86	30.2
Prior Stroke/ TIA / SE (%)	20	55	20
Parox. AF	33	17	15
CHF (%)	32	63	36
Baseline ASA (%)	39	36	39
VKA–Naïve (%)	50	38	43
Mean Follow-Up (yrs)	2.0	1,94	1.8
Lost to Follow-Up (%)	0.1	0,2	0.4

(e.g. to heparin) increases embolic risk. There are no published data on the peri-interventional use of factor Xa inhibitors undergoing pulmonary vein isolation. In an observational study using a by the manufacturer of dabigatran discouraged protocol, uninterrupted use of the drug except for the dose in the morning procedure (irrespective of renal function), monitored heparinization during the procedure

TABLE 7.3 Key differences in results of the three available randomized phase III trials comparing warfarin versus dabigatran (RE-LY) [5], rivaroxaban (ROCKET-AF) [6] and apixaban (ARISTOTLE) [7] in patients with non-valvular atrial fibrillation. Abbreviations: *D110* dabigatran 110 mg bid, *D150* dabigatran 150 mg bid, *ITT* intention to treat analysis, *NA* not available, *n.s.* non-significant, *OT* on treatment analysis, *RRR* relative risk reduction, *SSE* stroke and systemic embolism, *TTR* time in therapeutic range with warfarin

Key Differences			
	RELY®	ROCKET AF	ARISTOTLE
TTR	64.4%	55%	62.2%
SSE (RRR)	−35% (p<.001)	−12% ITT (n.s.) −21% OT (p<.02)	−21% (p=.011)
Ischemic stroke (RRR)	−24% (p=.03)	n.s.	n.s
Hemorrhagic Stroke (RRR)	−74% (p<.001)	−41% (p<.03)	−49% (p<.001)
Major Bleed (RRR)	D150 (n.s.) D110 −20% (p=.003)	n.s.	−21% (p<.001)
All cause mortality (RRR)	−12% (p=.051)	n.s.	−11% (p=.047)
Vascular death (RRR)	−15% (p=.04)	n.s.	NA
Permanent withdrawal (%)	21% (16% W)	23.7% (22.2% W)	25% (27% W)
Dosage/day	2	1	2

and reinitiation of dabigatran 0–3 h after sheath removal, increased the risk of bleeding and of embolic complications compared to uninterrupted VKA use [9]. However, at least four other studies [10–13] have shown that if a strategy of bridging and restarting of coagulation is appropriately executed, dabigatran does not shows any difference in efficacy or safety compared to warfarin [8]. In addition, an extensive review of periprocedural data and practical recommendations for the management of such situations is available, as well as the key scientific data on the use of NOACs in other situations (e.g. urgent surgical interventions o acute coronary syndromes) have been recently published [8].

Left Atrial Appendage Closure

Left atrial appendage (LAA) is considered the main (but not the only) site of thrombus formation and consequently the principal origin of thromboembolism. For those selected patients with high stroke risk and with contraindications for anticoagulation, and for those who suffer a stroke while on therapeutic OAC, percutaneous LAA occlusion is an alternative treatment option (class IIb, level B) [1]. Thus, in these patients LAA closure might be considered as alternative therapy to surgical excision which may be considered in patients undergoing open heart surgery (class IIb, level C) [1], although the excision did not effectively prevented stroke in randomized clinical studies [14].

Pharmacological Cardioversion

For AF of recent ($\leq$7 days) onset or occurring $\leq$3 days after cardiac surgery, a new intravenous antiarrhythmic drug (vernakalant), which blocks several ion channels but preferentially in the atria has been approved and added to recommended drug strategies [1]. Vernakalant has little impact on ventricular ion channels involved in repolarization. This drug has a rapid onset of action and a mean elimination half-life of 3–5 h. Conversion to sinus rhythm is achieved in approximately the half of patients with recent onset AF with a median conversion time of 8–14 min. Vernakalant should be administered as a 10 min-infusion of 3 mg/kg, and if AF persists after 15 min, a second infusion of 2 mg/kg can be given.

Vernakalant is contraindicated in patients with hypotension, recent (<30 days) acute coronary syndromes, NYHA class III and IV heart failure, severe aortic stenosis and QT prolongation (uncorrected QT >440 ms) and should be used with caution in patients with NYHA I o II heart failure because increased hypotension risk. In addition, it should not be used in patients with left ventricular ejection fraction of $\leq$35 %.

Thus, when pharmacological cardioversion is preferred in patients without or with minimal structural heart disease, intravenous flecainide, propafenone, ibutilide or vernakalant are actually recommended (class I, level A) [1]. In patients with AF ≤7 days and moderate structural heart disease, but without any of the mentioned contraindications, vernakalant may be considered but used with caution in patients with NYHA I and II heart failure (class IIb, level B). Furthermore, this drug may be also considered after cardiac surgery (≤3 days) for conversion of post-operative AF (class IIb, level B) but not for conversion of longer that 7 days lasting AF or for conversion of typical atrial flutter.

In conclusion, in emergent situations with haemodynamic instability electrical cardioversion is recommended. In elective situations electrical o pharmacological cardioversion may be attempted (depending of patient and physician choice). Those patients without structural heart disease may be pharmacologically treated with intravenous flecainide, propafenone and vernakalant as first choice and if it fails to revert the arrhythmia amiodarone can be used in a second step. Those patients with moderate structural heart disease may undergo first ibutilide (except if significant (≥14 mm) left ventricular hypertrophy is present) or vernakalant, and if fails also amiodarone can be used as second step. However, this last drug still remains the only pharmacological alternative for those patients with severe structural heart disease [1].

New Considerations of Antiarrhythmic Drugs for Prevention of AF

Antiarrhythmic drug therapy should be considered for those individuals with resistant symptoms due to recurrent AF. The safety-first principle should prevail because these drugs may induce adverse events and even mortality in some individuals. Thus, short-term (4 weeks post-cardioversion) therapy may be considered with flecainide since it is still effective (estimated at 80 % of the effect of long-term therapy) but not with amiodarone [1]. Thus, short-term therapy may be useful in patients with high risk of drug-induced adverse effects or with infrequent recurrences of AF (class IIb, level B).

As a consequence of the PALLAS trial [15], a significant modification of the recommendations for the use of antiarrhythmic drugs has been done [1]. Thus, dronedarone should not be used in patients with permanent AF (>6 months) or with significant cardiovascular disease burden. In addition, treatment should only be initiated and supervised by a specialist and monitoring of liver function tests is advisable in patients on long-term treatment. The concomitant use of dabigatran and dronedarone must be avoided because plasma concentrations of dabigatran are increased.

Importantly, dronedarone is contraindicated in patients with unstable haemodynamic conditions, with a history of (or current) heart failure or left ventricular dysfunction. Dronedarone is only recommended in patients with recurrent AF as a moderate effective antiarrhythmic drug for the maintenance of sinus rhythm who do not present a significant structural heart disease (class I, level A) but is not recommended in patients with permanent AF (class III, level B). Amiodarone still remains the best drug to prevent recurrences.

Further information of the unmet needs of antiarrhythmic drug therapy is detailed explained in other chapters of this book (see Martínez-Rubio et al.)

New Data of Ablation

Cather ablation may be a curative approach but it has the inherent risk of invasive procedures with possible major complications as stroke, tamponade, peripheral vascular complications, etc. Although catheter ablation seems more effective than antiarrhythmic drug therapy in maintaining sinus rhythm, long-term efficacy of the technique cannot be predicted in an individual basis and universal coverage is actually impossible. However, it may be a reasonable first-line strategy in selected patients (i.e. those with paroxysmal AF preferring interventional treatment with a low risk profile for procedure-associated complications or those patients with risk of drug-induced adverse effects). In addition, catheter ablation may be an alternative for those patients with recurrent symptoms under antiarrhythmic drug treatment who prefer further rhythm control therapy (class I, level A) and it should target isolation of the pulmonary veins (class IIa, level A). This invasive method may be considered as first-line therapy in selected patients with symptomatic paroxysmal AF considering patient choice, benefit and risk (class IIa, level B). When AF recurs within the first 6 weeks after catheter ablation, a watch-and-wait rhythm control therapy should be considered (class IIa, level B).

If VKA drugs are used, catheter ablation should be performed without interruption of anticoagulation, and later, it should not be interrupted in those patients at high-risk of stroke after apparent good results of the ablation procedure. Considerations of anticoagulation with NOACs during ablation have been previously commented in this chapter.

Surgical ablation seems more effective than catheter ablation but even with the cost of a higher complication rate (38). Therefore, it is a reserved technique for those very selected patients undergoing other concomitant surgical procedures such as aorto-coronary bypass or valve replacement.

Conclusions

AF remains a major clinical problem and, therefore, intensive research is undertaken which results in several new data of antiarrhythmic, as well as, preventive strategies of AF complications. Since thromboembolism (especially stroke) is one of the major complications of AF, several new data on risk stratification methodology and on pharmacological prevention of embolic complications and bleedings are undertaken. The NOACs open a new perspective in this setting with some still open questions, but with remarkable efficacy and safety data.

References

1. Camm AJ, Lip GYH, DeCaterina R, Savelieva I, Atar D, Hohnloser SH, Hindricks G, Kirchhof P. 2012 focused update of the ESC guidelines for the management of atrial fibrillation. Eur Heart J. 2012;33:2719–47.
2. Lip GY. Stroke in atrial fibrillation: epidemiology and thromboprophylaxis. J Thromb Haemost. 2011;9 Suppl 1:344–51.
3. Olesen JB, Lip GY, Hansen ML, Tolstrup JS, Lindhardsen J, Selmer C, Ahlehoff O, Olsen AM, Gislason GH, Torp-Pedersen C. Validation of risk stratification schemes for predicting stroke and thromboembolism in patients with atrial fibrillation: nationwide cohort study. BMJ. 2011;342:d124.
4. Friberg L, Rosenqvist M, Lip GY. Evaluation of risk stratification schemes for ischaemic stroke and bleeding in 182,678 patients with atrial fibrillation: the Swedish atrial fibrillation cohort study. Eur Heart J. 2012;33:1500–10.
5. Connolly SJ, Ezekowitz MD, Yusuf S, et al. Dabigatran versus warfarin in patients with atrial fibrillation. N Engl J Med. 2009;361:1139–51.
6. Patel MR, Mahaffey KW, Garg J, et al. Rivaroxaban versus warfarin in nonvalvular atrial fibrillation. N Engl J Med. 2011;365(10): 883–91.
7. Granger CB, Alexander JH, McMurray JJ, et al. Apixaban versus warfarin in patients with atrial fibrillation. N Engl J Med. 2011;365(11):981–92.
8. Heidbuchel H, Verhamme P, Alings M, Antz M, Hacke W, Oldgren J, Sinnaeve P, Camm AJ, Kirchhof P. European heart rhythm association practical guide on the use of new oral anticoagulants in patients with non-valvular atrial fibrillation. Europace. 2013;15:625–51.
9. Lakkireddy D, Reddy YM, Di Biase L, Vanga SR, Santangeli P, Swarup V, et al. Feasibility and safety of dabigatran versus warfarin for periprocedural anticoagulation in patients undergoing radiofrequency ablation for atrial fibrillation: results from a multicenter prospective registry. J Am Coll Cardiol. 2012;59:1168–74.
10. Kaseno K, Naito S, Nakamura K, Sakamoto T, Sasaki T, Tsukada N, et al. Efficacy and safety of periprocedural dabigatran in patients undergoing catheter ablation of atrial fibrillation. Circ J. 2012;76:2337–42.
11. Snipelisky D, Kauffman C, Prussak K, Johns G, Venkatachalam K, Kusumoto F. A comparison of bleeding complications post-ablation between warfarin and dabigatran. J Interv Card Electrophysiol. 2012;35:29–33.
12. Winkle RA, Mead RH, Engel G, Kong MH, Patrawala RA. The use of dabigatran immediately after atrial fibrillation ablation. J Cardiovasc Electrophysiol. 2012;23:264–8.

13. Kim JS, She F, Jongnarangsin K, Chugh A, Latchamsetty R, Ghanbari H, et al. Dabigatran vs warfarin for radiofrequency catheter ablation of atrial fibrillation. Heart Rhythm. 2013;10(4):483–9. doi:10.1016/j.hrthm.2012.12.011.

14. Lewalter T, Ibrahim R, Albers R, Camm AJ. An update and current expert opinions on percutaneous left atrial appendage occlusion for stroke prevention in atrial fibrillation. Europace. 2013;15:652–6.

15. Connolly SJ, Camm AJ, Halperin JL, Joyner C, Alings M, Amerena J, Atar D, Avezum A´, Blomstro¨MP, Borggrefe M, Budaj A, Chen SA, Ching CK, Commerford P, Dans A, Davy JM, Delacre´taz E, Di Pasquale G, Diaz R, Dorian P, Flaker G, Golitsyn S, Gonzalez-Hermosillo A, Granger CB, Heidbu¨chel H, Kautzner J, Kim JS, Lanas F, Lewis BS, Merino JL, Morillo C, Murin J, Narasimhan C, Paolasso E, Parkhomenko A, Peters NS, Sim KH, Stiles MK, Tanomsup S, Toivonen L, Tomcsa´nyi J, Torp-Pedersen C, Tse HF, Vardas P, Vinereanu D, Xavier D, Zhu J, Zhu JR, Baret-Cormel L, Weinling E, Staiger C, Yusuf S, Chrolavicius S, Afzal R, Hohnloser SH; PALLAS Investigators. Dronedarone in high-risk permanent atrial fibrillation. N Engl J Med. 2011;365:2268–76.

Index

G.-A. Dan et al. (eds.), *Atrial Fibrillation Therapy*, Current
Cardiovascular Therapy, DOI 10.1007/978-1-4471-5475-4,
© Springer-Verlag London 2014

Printed by Printforce, the Netherlands